I0837407

The FRUCTOSE FREE COOKBOOK

A COMPREHENSIVE DIET GUIDE AND COOKBOOK WITH OVER 120 DELICIOUS RECIPES FOR PEOPLE WITH FRUCTOSE INTOLERANCE OR MALABSORPTION

MONET MANBACCI, PH.D.

(Edition-1)

Copyright © 2020 by Monet Manbacci.

All Right Reserved.

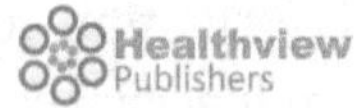

Disclaimer Notice

No part of this publication may be reproduced, distributed, or transmitted in any form or by any means, including photocopying, recording, or other electronic or mechanical methods, or by any information storage and retrieval system without the prior written permission of the publisher, except in the case of very brief quotations embodied in critical reviews and certain other noncommercial uses permitted by copyright law.

Please, consider that the information in this book is only for educational purposes. No warranties of any kind are implied or declared in this book. Readers acknowledge that the author of this book is not engaged in the rendering of medical, legal, financial, or professional advice. Hence, consult a licensed professional before applying any hints or techniques outlined in this book. By reading this notice, the readers agree that the author of this book is not responsible for any direct or indirect losses that are incurred because of the use of the information contained in this book, including but not limited to inaccuracies, omissions, and errors.

This book has been published by the Healthview Publishers. All rights reserved.

Table of Contents

INTRODUCTION

Fructose intolerance (FI) mostly observes in people with irritable bowel syndrome (IBS) or other GI disorders. In such patients, fructose is not digested or absorbed well in the gastrointestinal system, causing abdominal pain, bloating, gas, diarrhea, and nausea in some cases.

If you or your loved one has been diagnosed with Fructose Intolerance, you already know how hard this intolerance could be and how tough it can be managed. Research studies have found that many issues come from the followings:

- Not knowing much about the intolerance
- Self-treatment
- Ignoring signs and symptoms
- Not knowing about triggering foods to avoid
- Mismanagement of the disorder
- Not following the doctor's orders correctly or completely

One of the best ways to manage your symptoms, and have a healthier life, is to follow a "Fructose Free" or a "Low Fructose" diet, with the help of a comprehensive diet guide and cookbook.

This book gives the readers valuable information about healthy nutritional choices, foods to eat or to avoid, food preparation, meal planning, and how to create biweekly cooking plans for fructose intolerants. It primarily provide readers with necessary nutritional information about the condition and then, guide readers on their fructose free cooking and dietary plans. This book is recommended to the groups below:

1. You are fructose intolerant and want to know how to manage your diet, how to cook varieties of foods, and how to balance your meals using effective meal plans.
2. You have a fructose intolerant family member and want to know how to prepare low fructose meals or make meal plans.
3. You recently realized that you are fructose intolerant and do not know how to cook for yourself
4. Your loved one newly diagnosed with a fructose intolerant disorder.

If you have recently diagnosed or if your loved one have recently diagnosed, this book is an excellent source for you to take initial necessary dietary steps, learn how to cook varieties of low fructose foods, how to manage your disorder, how to do meal planning and learn about diet tips.

If you have this disorder for a long period, the information in this book can also help you maintain your remission periods and balance your life with fructose free recipes better than before.

Fructose can certainly cause issues when it comes to choosing what you eat and drink. Not only does the condition cause digestive tract irritation and uncomfortable symptoms, but long-term consequences may include malnutrition. To make matters more complicated, your dietary habits may worsen symptoms. Eating and avoiding certain foods explained in this book can help prevent symptom flares. That is why one of the chapters of this book focuses on food preparation and meal planning.

Comprehensive lists of foods to avoid and foods to eat are presented in this book as well. The book then fully covers how to cook for fructose intolerants following by more than

120 cooking recipes. This chapter covers various types of recipes for breakfast, appetizers, soups, salads, snacks, main courses, desserts, and drinks. Each recipe starts with a brief explanation, preparation time, cooking time, total time, ingredients, instructions, cooking tips, Fructose Intolerance-related tips, and nutrition facts.

The nutrition facts of the recipes in this book have been analyzed by "Verywell fit" Recipe Nutrition Calculator (Ref: https://www.verywellfit.com). Biweekly cooking plan samples are given to you in Chapter 4. The same chapter provides you with blank biweekly cooking plan tables for you to write your cooking plan and stick it to your fridge.

It has to be reminded that the recommendations, hints, and tips provided in this book have been gathered from various related research studies and references from different online/offline resources. These have been found useful by the author of this book, but it does not mean that all will work for you or for your loved one. It should be understood that any recommendations or tips in this book can only be followed only when you take responsibility for it. Be sure that you always talk to your doctor or dietician about the recipes, steps, or hints this book recommends to make sure that they are in line with your health condition.

CHAPTER 1: COMPREHENSIVE LISTS OF FOODS TO EAT & TO AVOID

This chapter presents foods to eat, foods to consume in moderation and foods to fully avoid for people with fructose intolerance. It has to be noted that most of the items in the lists has been found from the reference below: https://www.healthhype.com/nutrition-guide-for-fructose-malabsorption.html

Fruits to avoid

Apples (all types), cherries, figs, grapes (black), guava, honeydew melon, lychee, mango, nashi fruit, papaya, pears, dates, persimmon, plumes, prunes, raisins, star fruit, sultana, quince, watermelon. Dried fruits, fruit compotes and jams in general. | R

Fruits to consume

Grapefruit, lemons, cumquat, limes | G

Fruits to consume in Moderation

Avocado, bananas, passion fruit, pineapple, rhubarb, strawberries, raspberries, blackberries, boysenberries, blueberries, cantaloupes, cranberries, white grapes, jack-fruit, kiwi, mandarins, oranges, tangelo, apricots, nectarines, peaches | M

Vegetables to avoid

Artichoke, eggplant, green peppers, green cabbage, kale, leeks, lettuce (iceberg), pickles (e.g. sweet cucumbers), radishes, squash, tomatoes, turnips, watercress. | R

Vegetables to consume

Bouillon, celery, escarole, hash-browns, mustard greens, pea pods (immature), potatoes (white), pumpkin, shallots, spinach, Swiss chard. | G

Vegetables to consume in Moderation

Asparagus, beets, carrots, dandelion greens, cauliflower, endive, legumes (beans, peas, lentils), lettuce, mushrooms, onions, green onions, soy, sweet potatoes, turnip greens, zucchini. | M

Sugars and Sweeteners to avoid

Agave syrup (in tequila, margaritas, soft drinks), caramel, rock sugar, corn syrup solids, **fructose**, fruit juice concentrate, golden syrup (cane syrup), **High Fructose Corn Syrup (HFCS), honey**, invert sugar, licorice, molasses, raw sugar, palm sugar, sweets >50g, soft drinks with sucrose >375 mL.
Sugar substitutes: HSH, sorbitol, stevia, and sucralose.

Sugars and Sweeteners to consume

Acesulfam potassium, dextrin, erythritol, glucose: dextrose, glucodin, glycogen, maltodextrin: modified starch, moducal, trehalose.

Sugars and Sweeteners to consume in Moderation

Barley malt syrup, brown rice syrup, **brown sugar**, corn syrup (with no added fructose), **maple syrup**, sorghum syrup, grape syrup, sucrose (white or cane sugar).
Sugar substitutes: dulcitol, isomalt, lactalol, lacticol, litesse, lycasin, maltitol, mannitol, saccharin, sucanat, trimoline, xylitol.

Breads and Cereals to avoid

Brown rice, sweetened breakfast cereals or with raisins, honey.

Breads and Cereals to consume

Barley, breads and pasta without fructose or gluten-free, wheat-free rye bread, corn meal, cornflakes (non-flavored), grits, grouts, oatmeal, porridge (cooked oatmeal), plain muffins, rice (white), rice or buckwheat noodles, rye flour, tortilla

Breads and Cereals to consume in Moderation

Wheat: dinkle, kamut, sourdoughs, spelt, whole meal and wheat products: biscuits, noodles, pasta, and pastry.

Proteins to avoid

Meat, fish: if processed, sweetened, or commercially breaded, coconut milk or coconut cream.

Proteins to consume

Meat: fresh, not commercially breaded, fish: fresh or tinned without sauce, other seafood, **eggs, grains, nuts, seeds**: amaranth, flaxseed, millet, poppy, pistachios, sesame, tahini, sunflower

Proteins to consume in Moderation

Legumes: chick peas, lentils, lima, mung, soy (including tofu), Nuts

Dairy to avoid

Sweetened milk products, ice creams.	R

Dairy to consume

Plain, unsweetened milk, yogurt, cheese.	G

Sauces and Spices to avoid

Sauces: Barbeque's, Sweet&Sour, Hot mustard, chutney, ketchup, relish, soy sauce, vinegar: apple cider, balsamic. **Spices:** chervil, dill weed, ginger, hot chili pepper, pumpkin pie seasoning.	R

Sauces and Spices to consume

Basil, bay, cinnamon, cumin, curry, marjoram, oregano, parsley, rosemary, thyme.	G

Sauce and Spices to Consume in Moderation

Distilled vinegar. Coriander, garlic, onions, parsnip, spring onions.	M

Drinks to avoid

Fruit juices: apple, apricot, mango, orange, pear, peach, prune, sweat cherry, soft drinks with sorbitol or HFCS; **alcohol:** except dry white wine, powdered sweetened beverages, sweetened milk/vegetable/soy drinks, coffee substitutes with chicory.	R

Drinks to consume

Water: tap water, non-flavored bottled water, mineral water, **tea, coffee:** not chicory based coffee substitutes.	G

Drinks to Consume in Moderation

Fruit juices: blackberry, cranberry, white grapes; Alcohol: dry white or red wine (one glass per serving).	M

Important Note-1: People with fructose intolerance who cannot tolerate wheat products (gluten) such as white bread, pasta, and breakfast cereals might have issues with artichokes, asparagus, radish, spring onions, and anything with chicory.

Important Note-2: People with fructose intolerance who cannot tolerate beans might find other legumes such as peas, soy, lentils, broccoli, Brussel's sprouts, cabbage, cauliflower, kale, turnip greens, and whole grains intolerable as well.

Important Notes-3:

- Cooking vegetables like carrots can make higher fructose than consuming them raw. Try not to cook carrots a lot.
- Remember that the whole-grain bread with gluten has more fructose than refined bread.
- Typically, brown rice has more fructose than white rice.
- Fresh potatoes have more fructose than old ones.
- Medications such as vitamins and supplements, may contain fructose or sorbitol. It is recommended to always check the labels and purchased medications with no fructose.

Important Note-4: Remember that the lists above are the general lists of foods to eat and to avoid. You may find some foods to eat in the list that you cannot tolerate well or vice versa. Always try to check your tolerance levels regarding each item. Then, write and remember your triggering foods to avoid.

This book tries its best to stick to the non-triggering foods presented in this chapter. However, you may need to do your minor adjustments to the recipes based on the foods you can tolerate.

CHAPTER 2. FOOD PREPARATION & MEAL PLANNING

The following tips can help you to have an effective food preparation and meal planning:

EATING HABITS

1- Eat smaller portions, but frequent meals 5 to 6 times a day.

2- Avoid any foods or drinks with lots of fructose explained in the previous chapter.

3- Keep yourself hydrated. Drink plenty of water and other allowed juices during a day. Pump-up your electrolyte intake, especially during flares using low-sugar sports drinks or use yours at home.

4- Drink slowly and chew well.

5- Do not use straw as you may ingest air, which can cause producing gas.

6- You can drink recommended herbal teas after your meal for better digestion, especially if you think that you ate a lot of your meal was heavy for you.

7- Give time to your herbal tea to brew well.

8- Eat your meal in peace and comfort in a relaxed place. Do not talk too much when you are eating your meal.

9- Do not work with your phone or laptop while eating your meals.

10- Do not drink water in the middle of eating meals.

11- Do not skip your breakfast at all.

12- Do not starve yourself. Determine right specific times for your meals and stick to those times.

13- Do not eat very late. Eat dinner at least 2 hours before your sleep time, or 3 to 4 hours after your lunch.

14- Always have a meal plan and follow it. The worst thing for you is not knowing what to eat and what to cook.

15- Reduce consuming alcohol, sugar, and caffeinated drink. Avoid consuming them in flare-up periods.

16- Do not leave your foods at normal temperature for more than 2 hours.

GROCERY SHOPPING

1- To prepare your meals in advance, you need to create a list before you go to the supermarket for daily or weekly shopping.

2- The list should include ingredients you need for your daily or weekly cooking plan. Remember that the ingredients should be well-tolerated.

3- Always try to purchase organic, non-GMO ingredients

4- Always try to buy lower-fat options.

5- For eggs, try to purchase organic, free-range types

6- For meat or pork, try to pick low-fat lean cuts

7- For poultry, skin-removed breasts and legs are the best options.

8- For cheese, try to purchase low-fat lactose-free options. Use cheese in moderation.

9- For milk and yogurts, always purchase unsweetened and unflavored types.

10- For milk, try to purchase low-fat lactose-free options such as almond milk or rice milk. Use milk in moderation.

11- For grains, try not to get whole-wheat or whole-grain options. Stick to gluten-free options. White breads may also work for you.

12- For bread, try to find gluten-free bread that is not highly processed.

13- For baking, purchase gluten-free flours such as almond flour.

14- Purchase fruits and vegetables that you can tolerate well.

15- For oil, purchase extra virgin olive oil or avocado oil. Avoid coconut oil.

16- Keep having turmeric, and cinnamon in your kitchen cabinet.

17- Avoid purchasing processed foods.

18- For sauces such as mayonnaise, try to purchase organic low fat and low sodium types. Avoid ketchup.

19- For beef, chicken, or vegetable broth, try to buy organic low sodium types.

20- Always purchase organic potatoes.

21- It is not recommended to purchase fruit juices with added sugar, and juices from concentrate. The best option for you is to make a juice from non-triggering fruits at home.

22- If you want to purchase almond butter, get the organic and smooth one.

23- To make your meals sweet, brown sugar might be a great option.

24- Maple syrup in limited amount (1 tbsp) may work for you as a sweetener option.

25- Try to purchase fresh foods instead of frozen or canned foods.

26- Read the ingredients of the snacks you may want to purchase. Make sure you can tolerate all ingredients well.

27- Fully avoid consuming products with high fructose or with High Fructose Corn Syrup (HFCS).

COOKING TOOLS

You do not necessarily need to buy any specific tools to cook for a person with fructose intolerance, but here are some tools that can help you ease the cooking process:

1- <u>Cast Iron skillet:</u> some people suggest having an iron skillet to absorb iron better.
2- <u>Blender:</u> for those who can use nuts in moderation, they need to blend them well. Having a suitable blender/mixer can help you cook well-blended meals such as soups, smoothies, nut butter, and juices.
3- <u>Juicer:</u> having a powerful juicer can help you taking the juices of fruits and vegetables. With this tool, you may have fruits or vegetables that cannot be tolerated because of having high insoluble fiber.
4- <u>Small lunch-dinner boxes:</u> it is recommended for people with fructose intolerance to eat smaller portions six times a day. One great idea to follow this eating style is to provide lunch, snacks, and dinners in separate boxes. For instance, you can put your lunch in two small lunch boxes instead of a big one, and eat each box in different time (e.g., with two hours of time-difference) at your workplace.
5- <u>Spiralizer:</u> to have spaghetti-like zucchini, potatoes, and pumpkin, you may need to have a spiralizer.
6- <u>Air fryer:</u> air frying can be a great cooking option, as it does not need much oil. You can make great zucchini or potato chip snacks or other meals using an air fryer.

7- <u>Timer and thermometer:</u> both are helpful tools for you to cook delicious meals. Remember that meats should be cooked well. Hence, you can use these tools to check if inside meats cooked well or not.

KITCHEN PREPARATION

Here are some of the tips to prepare the kitchen and yourself before cooking:

1. Wash your hands perfectly when you want to cook.
2. Always wash fruits and vegetables before using them.
3. Remember to use allowed skin-removed or poached fruits.
4. Remember not to consume fruit cores or vegetable seeds a lot.
5. Wash meats before cooking. Use disposable gloves when washing meats and put gloves in the garbage after. Always wash your hands with warm water right after washing meats and poultries.
6. Use a separate cutting board for raw meat
7. Keep raw meats away from other foods in the kitchen and fridge.
8. Never mix cooked foods with raw meats. Mixing can happen in plates, cutting boards, etc. Never eat such foods.
9. Remember to cook or boil meats, seafood, and vegetables in perfection.
10. Keep the kitchen area well-cleaned and sanitized.

MEAL PLANNING

1- Use proper cooking methods explained in this book. Keep your cooking style simple:

a. If you are in remission (it seems that your symptoms are gone for couple of weeks), you are free to apply cooking techniques such as stir-fry foods in moderation with extra virgin olive oil.

b. If you are in a flare, try to stick to techniques such as boiling, steaming, and poaching.

c. Grating spices such as ginseng is better than consuming ginseng powders.

2- You should have your meal plans ready. Use the information on this book to create your meal plans. The plans should include only foods that you can consume.

3- You also should know the strategy of finding triggering foods for yourself. To keep it simple, if you ate a specific food at any time and observed any symptoms such as diarrhea, cramping, gas, bloating, and abdominal pain, you might be intolerant to that particular food. If you ate a meal and you are not sure about the ingredient(s) you are intolerant inside, you have to write this meal in your journal and record your symptoms and conditions there. Then, you need to review your journal at the end of each week or two again and check if you can find any relations or common ingredient(s) between different meals you could not tolerate or not. You can visit a dietitian or a nutritionist to guide you more on how to find triggering foods.

4- Create at least two, two-week meal plans, with enough variety and stick to them according to your health condition. Your meal plan should have the following cooking/eating items:

a. Meal-1: Breakfast

b. Meal-2: Snack

   c.   Meal-3: Lunch-1

   d.   Meal-4: Lunch-2

   e.   Meal-5: Snack

   f.   Meal-6: Dinner

   g.   Eight glasses of drinks

Soup, salad, appetizer, and dessert options should be added to your schedules as well. Chapter 4 of this book presents two detailed examples of biweekly meal plans. After the examples, this book gives you two blank meal plans. You can fill the blanked spaces to design your own biweekly meal plan.

5- If you are working outside the home, plan to cook for your next day's lunch at work.

6- Prepare or purchase a journal designed explicitly for people with fructose intolerance to keep the records of your meals taken and symptoms you experience.

OTHER TIPS

1- As an advanced technique, you can prepare different meal plans for different seasons, which can help you use fresh seasonal ingredients in your meals.

2- This book helps you cooking fast and easy delicious fructose free meals. However, allocate time as much as you can for your cooking.

   a.   Presentation is very important to increase the appetite. If you see cooking as an art, you can definitely prepare meals with an excellent presentation based on your artistic and creative ideas.

   b.   Try to have colorful meals that can increase your appetite, as well. Have your main course with colorful sides such as green (zucchinis), orange (carrots), yellow (lemon wedges or potatoes), etc.

c. Be creative: by reading this book and your hard work on finding the best tolerable foods, you will learn which ingredients are great, which are safe, and which are not okay. Then, you can create your meals or judge any meal recipes based on your knowledge.

3- Using alkaline water: there are not so many scientific studies about the impact of using alkaline waters on fructose intolerant patients. However, some found that the alkaline water (known as Kangen water in some references) could reduce their symptoms, and they had longer remission periods. Other properties of alkaline-water machines might also be helpful. For example, alkaline water machines typically produce waters with low pH (e.g., 2.5 pH) that possibly remove pesticides from the skin of foods such as fruits, vegetables, and rice (if you wash them with such waters). Hence, consuming alkaline water might be an option for you to investigate.

CHAPTER 3. LOW FRUCTOSE COOKING RECIPES

This chapter provides you with more than 120 fantastic delicious cooking recipes for people with fructose intolerance. It consists of various recipes to cook, serve, and enjoy, such as breakfasts, soups, salads, appetizers, main courses for lunch and dinner, desserts, drinks, and snacks.

Each cooking recipe starts with a brief introduction, preparation time, cooking time, total time, serving size, ingredients, instructions, cooking tips, Fructose Intolerance (FI)-related tips, and nutrition facts. It has to be noted that the nutrition facts of the recipes in this book have been analyzed by "Verywell fit" Recipe Nutrition Calculator.

BREAKFASTS

GLUTEN-FREE FLUFFY PANCAKE

A great gluten-free pancake for those who cannot tolerate gluten. You can make this great pancake if you are lactose-intolerant, as well.

- Prep Time: 5 minutes
- Cook Time: 10 minutes
- Total Time: 15 minutes
- Serving: 4

<u>Ingredients:</u>

- 2 organic, free-range eggs
- 2 cups white rice flour or almond flour

- 2 cups lactose-free milk with one tablespoon lemon juice
- 1 teaspoon lime juice
- 1.5 tablespoon baking powder
- Salt to taste

<u>Instructions</u>

1. In a medium bowl, mix and whisk all ingredients.
2. Heat a large pan with extra virgin olive oil and cook both sides of pancakes until golden over medium heat.
3. Enjoy!

<u>Cooking Tips:</u>

- You can pour maple syrup (1 tbsp) on top of your pancakes if you can tolerate maple syrup.

Nutrition Facts

Servings: 4

Amount per serving

Calories	402
	% Daily Value*
Total Fat 7.3g	9%
Saturated Fat 3.5g	17%
Cholesterol 97mg	32%
Sodium 132mg	6%
Total Carbohydrate 71.2g	26%
Dietary Fiber 3.4g	12%
Total Sugars 6.3g	
Protein 11.5g	
Vitamin D 8mcg	39%
Calcium 20mg	2%
Iron 1mg	4%
Potassium 93mg	2%

Eggs, Salmon, and Avocado

This breakfast contains a great source of healthy fats and protein. A smooth, fast, and delicious breakfast recipe to cook!

- Prep Time: 5 minutes
- Cook Time: 10 minutes
- Total Time: 15 minutes
- Serving: 2

<u>Ingredients:</u>

- 2 scrambled eggs
- 2 oz salmon, cooked or canned
- ½ avocado
- 1 teaspoon extra virgin olive oil

<u>Instructions</u>

1. Heat a large pan with high-quality extra virgin olive oil and scramble your eggs over medium heat.
2. Mix your scramble with avocado cubes and small salmon pieces. Enjoy!

<u>Cooking Tips:</u>

- You can also mash your avocado instead of cubing it.

Nutrition Facts

Servings: 2

Amount per serving

Calories	353
	% Daily Value*
Total Fat 30.4g	39%
Saturated Fat 6.7g	34%
Cholesterol 182mg	61%
Sodium 107mg	5%
Total Carbohydrate 9.6g	3%
Dietary Fiber 6.7g	24%
Total Sugars 1.4g	
Protein 13.5g	
Vitamin D 44mcg	220%
Calcium 26mg	2%
Iron 2mg	9%
Potassium 677mg	14%

BAKED PINEAPPLE

For those who have fructose intolerance, cooked, and unsweet fruits are great breakfast ingredients.

- Prep Time: 5 minutes
- Cook Time: 30 minutes
- Total Time: 35 minutes
- Serving: 2

Ingredients

- 1 teaspoon cinnamon
- 1 teaspoon extra virgin olive oil
- 2 cups of water
- 1 tablespoon maple syrup
- ½ pineapple

Instructions

1. In a medium/large pot, boil pineapple with cinnamon, olive oil, water, and maple syrup over high heat for 30 minutes.
2. Enjoy!

Nutrition Facts

Servings: 2

Amount per serving	
Calories	**173**
	% Daily Value*
Total Fat 2.7g	4%
Saturated Fat 0.3g	2%
Cholesterol 0mg	0%
Sodium 12mg	1%
Total Carbohydrate 40.6g	15%
Dietary Fiber 6g	21%
Total Sugars 32g	
Protein 0.7g	
Vitamin D 0mcg	0%
Calcium 27mg	2%
Iron 1mg	6%
Potassium 258mg	5%

PINEAPPLE OATMEAL BARS

As oatmeal has lots of soluble fiber, it is a good option for fructose intolerance people. It's typically mild and colon-friendly. This bar is gluten and lactose-free with a great taste of banana and ginseng.

- Prep Time: 10 minutes
- Cook Time: 25 minutes
- Total Time: 35 minutes
- Serving: 4

<u>Ingredients</u>

- 1 organic pineapple
- 1 teaspoon ground ginseng
- ½ teaspoon salt
- ½ cup organic smooth almond butter
- 2 teaspoons pure vanilla extract
- 2 teaspoons ground cinnamon
- ¾ teaspoon baking powder
- ¾ cup gluten-free flour
- ½ cup rolled oats (or a small package of ready oatmeal)

<u>Instructions</u>

1. Preheat oven to 375 °F.
2. Cook the pineapple or use a pineapple compote.
3. Mix your pineapple with salt, almond butter, ginseng, vanilla extract, cinnamon, baking powder, flour, and oats.
4. Pour your mix into a suitable oven pan.
5. Bake your oatmeal for 25 minutes until inside cooks well. Cut the baked oatmeal like bars.
6. Let it be cooled first and then serve!

Cooking Tips:

- It is recommended to use organic oatmeal.
- To check if the inside cooks well, insert a toothpick inside. If it comes out without sticking to your bar, it shows that it cooked well.

Fructose Intolerance-related Tips:

- Reduce your monthly oatmeal intakes if you found this recipe irritative to your gut.

Nutrition Facts

Servings: 4

Amount per serving

Calories	612
	% Daily Value*
Total Fat 34.2g	44%
Saturated Fat 3.4g	17%
Cholesterol 0mg	0%
Sodium 296mg	13%
Total Carbohydrate 70g	25%
Dietary Fiber 18.2g	65%
Total Sugars 27.9g	
Protein 14.5g	
Vitamin D 0mcg	0%
Calcium 249mg	19%
Iron 4mg	23%
Potassium 931mg	20%

AVOCADO & EGG BREAKFAST TOAST

A very simple, delicious breakfast dish, high in protein and healthy fat.

- Prep Time: 5 minutes
- Cook Time: 10 minutes
- Total Time: 15 minutes
- Serving: 2

Ingredients

- 4 slices of white toast or gluten-free bread
- ½ cup low fat lactose-free Havarti cheese

- ½ avocado
- 2 large organic free-range eggs
- 4 egg whites
- 1 tablespoon lime juice
- Salt and pepper to taste

Instructions

1. Toast your white bread toasts the way you want.
2. Mix cheese, eggs, egg whites, salt, and pepper in a bowl and scramble it in a pan over medium heat for 7 minutes.
3. Coat your toasts with scrambled mix and mashed avocado. Then, squeeze lime. Enjoy!

Cooking Tips:

- You can use low-fat lactose-free feta cheese instead of Havarti, as well.

Nutrition Facts	
Servings: 2	
Amount per serving	
Calories	**411**
	% Daily Value*
Total Fat 26.4g	34%
Saturated Fat 6.5g	32%
Cholesterol 191mg	64%
Sodium 467mg	20%
Total Carbohydrate 21.2g	8%
Dietary Fiber 7.2g	26%
Total Sugars 2.5g	
Protein 24.7g	
Vitamin D 18mcg	88%
Calcium 103mg	8%
Iron 2mg	12%
Potassium 751mg	16%

Smoothie Bowl

A mix of skin-removed and chopped fruits can create a tremendous rich breakfast!

- Prep Time: 10 minutes
- Cook Time: 0 minutes
- Total Time: 10 minutes
- Serving: 2

Ingredients

- 1 banana, sliced
- 1 cup almond milk or lactose-free milk
- 1 cup pineapple chunks
- 1 cup diced cantaloupe

Instructions

1. Blend all mentioned ingredients in a blender. Serve and Enjoy!

Cooking Tips:

- You can use the same instruction to make fruit bowls with other fruits you can tolerate.
- You can add 1 cup of papaya to your bowl as well.

Nutrition Facts

Servings: 2

Amount per serving	
Calories	**419**
	% Daily Value*
Total Fat 29.2g	37%
Saturated Fat 25.5g	128%
Cholesterol 0mg	0%
Sodium 20mg	1%
Total Carbohydrate 43.3g	16%
Dietary Fiber 6.6g	24%
Total Sugars 30.6g	
Protein 4.5g	
Vitamin D 0mcg	0%
Calcium 42mg	3%
Iron 2mg	14%
Potassium 755mg	16%

ZUCCHINI BREAD OATMEAL

Enjoy the taste of grated zucchini and oatmeal and have a healthy fructose intolerance adapted breakfast!

- Prep Time: 5 minutes
- Cook Time: 7 minutes
- Total Time: 12 minutes
- Serving: 2

<u>Ingredients</u>

- ⅓ cup organic rolled oats or ready oatmeal
- 1 cup unsweetened almond or lactose-free milk
- ½ teaspoon cinnamon powder
- ½ cup zucchini
- 1 teaspoon vanilla extract
- 1 teaspoon brown sugar

<u>Instructions</u>

1. Mix your milk with cinnamon and oat in a medium pot and boil the mixture over medium heat for 4 minutes.
2. Grate zucchini, add it to the mix, and stir well for three minutes.
3. In a small bowl, mix vanilla extract and brown sugar.
4. When oatmeal cooked, remove from heat and pour the syrup on it.
5. Let it be cooled and then serve!

<u>Cooking Tips:</u>

- You can use 1tbsp maple syrup in this recipe if you can tolerate.

Nutrition Facts	
Servings: 2	
Amount per serving	
Calories	**82**
	% Daily Value*
Total Fat 2.7g	3%
Saturated Fat 0.3g	2%
Cholesterol 0mg	0%
Sodium 94mg	4%
Total Carbohydrate 11.5g	4%
Dietary Fiber 2.2g	8%
Total Sugars 0.9g	
Protein 2.6g	
Vitamin D 1mcg	3%
Calcium 162mg	12%
Iron 1mg	6%
Potassium 222mg	5%

BREAKFAST FRUIT SALAD

A mix of a variety of fruits (skin-removed and chopped) can create an excellent breakfast salad!

- Prep Time: 5 minutes
- Cook Time: 25 minutes
- Total Time: 30 minutes
- Serving: 6

Ingredients

- 1 can pineapple chunks
- 1 large firm banana, cubed
- 1 medium cantaloupe, skin removed and cubed
- 1 medium papaya, skin-removed and cubed
- 1 tablespoon lemon juice
- 1 tablespoon brown sugar (optional)
- ⅓ cup orange juice (optional)

Instructions

1. Mix all fruits in a bowl.

2. Boil your orange juice, lemon juice, and brown sugar in a small pot (over high heat). Stir well.

3. Let the juice be cooled. Then, add your cooled juice to the fruit bowl. Enjoy!

<u>Cooking Tips:</u>

- You can use orange juice in this recipe if you can tolerate it.

Nutrition Facts

Servings: 6

Amount per serving	
Calories	**108**
	% Daily Value*
Total Fat 0.4g	1%
Saturated Fat 0.1g	1%
Cholesterol 0mg	0%
Sodium 6mg	0%
Total Carbohydrate 27.7g	10%
Dietary Fiber 3.5g	13%
Total Sugars 18.8g	
Protein 1g	
Vitamin D 0mcg	0%
Calcium 17mg	1%
Iron 1mg	3%
Potassium 331mg	7%

BANANA SPLIT OATMEAL

A great combination of oatmeal and banana can make a great breakfast full of fiber and potassium.

- Prep Time: 10 minutes
- Cook Time: 0 minutes
- Total Time: 10 minutes
- Serving: 2

<u>Ingredients</u>

- ½ cup water, almond milk or lactose-free milk
- 1 cup old-fashioned rolled oats or a small ready oatmeal package

- ½ banana, cubed
- Salt to taste

<u>Instructions</u>

1. Boil your milk or water in a pot over high heat.
2. Add oat and salt to it. Stir for two more minutes.
3. Serve your oatmeal with cubed bananas. Enjoy!

<u>Cooking Tips:</u>

- You can use maple syrup in this recipe if you can tolerate.

Nutrition Facts

Servings: 2

Amount per serving	
Calories	**319**
	% Daily Value*
Total Fat 17.1g	22%
Saturated Fat 13.2g	66%
Cholesterol 0mg	0%
Sodium 89mg	4%
Total Carbohydrate 37.8g	14%
Dietary Fiber 6.2g	22%
Total Sugars 6g	
Protein 7.1g	
Vitamin D 0mcg	0%
Calcium 32mg	2%
Iron 3mg	16%
Potassium 412mg	9%

EGG TACOS WITH AVOCADO

Enjoy a breakfast sandwich with egg and avocado, which is full of healthy fats and functional proteins.

- Prep Time: 5 minutes
- Cook Time: 10 minutes
- Total Time: 15 minutes
- Serving: 2

<u>Ingredients</u>

- 4 small gluten-free tortillas
- 2 organic, free-range eggs
- ½ avocado
- Salt to taste

Instructions

1. Warm or toast tortillas.
2. Scramble or boil your eggs using salt.
3. Mash your avocado
4. Fill your tortillas with avocado and eggs. Enjoy!

Cooking Tips:

- You can use gluten-free bread (if you can tolerate them) instead of tortillas.

Nutrition Facts

Servings: 2

Amount per serving

Calories	373
	% Daily Value*
Total Fat 25.3g	32%
Saturated Fat 5.7g	29%
Cholesterol 164mg	55%
Sodium 167mg	7%
Total Carbohydrate 30.4g	11%
Dietary Fiber 9.8g	35%
Total Sugars 1.3g	
Protein 10.2g	
Vitamin D 15mcg	77%
Calcium 74mg	6%
Iron 2mg	11%
Potassium 636mg	14%

CRISPY HASH BROWN WITH EGG

Start your day with hash brown and egg! A great combination, as always!

- Prep Time: 20 minutes
- Cook Time: 15 minutes
- Total Time: 35 minutes

- Serving: 2

Ingredients

- 2 large yellow potatoes, shredded
- ¼ cup gluten-free flour
- 2 tablespoons extra virgin olive oil
- 2 organic range-free eggs
- Salt and pepper to taste

Instructions

1. Shred potatoes and rinse them until the water cleared. Dry potatoes.
2. Mix your potatoes with flour, eggs, salt, and pepper.
3. Flatten your mix in a large skillet and let it cook over medium heat until golden brown. Flip and cook the other side.
4. Remove from the skillet and drain with a paper towel. Enjoy!

Cooking Tips:

- To flip it quickly, you can cut in half or quarter.

Nutrition Facts

Servings: 2

Amount per serving

Calories	385
	% Daily Value*
Total Fat 18.7g	24%
Saturated Fat 3.4g	17%
Cholesterol 164mg	55%
Sodium 70mg	3%
Total Carbohydrate 45.9g	17%
Dietary Fiber 2.8g	10%
Total Sugars 3g	
Protein 10.2g	
Vitamin D 15mcg	77%
Calcium 34mg	3%
Iron 2mg	12%
Potassium 686mg	15%

Grilled Almond Butter Banana Sandwich

An excellent easy to make a sandwich for your breakfast.

- Prep Time: 5 minutes
- Cook Time: 0 minutes
- Total Time: 5 minutes
- Serving: 2

Ingredients

- 1 tablespoon extra virgin olive oil
- Few grams of almond butter
- 1 banana
- 4 slices of gluten-free bread
- Brown sugar (1 tbsp.)

Instructions

- Toast your bread slices, as you desired.
- Mash banana, coat your bread with banana, almond butter, and brown sugar. Enjoy!

Nutrition Facts

Servings: 2

Amount per serving

Calories	172
	% Daily Value*
Total Fat 8.7g	11%
Saturated Fat 1.3g	6%
Cholesterol 0mg	0%
Sodium 123mg	5%
Total Carbohydrate 23.3g	8%
Dietary Fiber 2.1g	8%
Total Sugars 8.4g	
Protein 2.4g	
Vitamin D 0mcg	0%
Calcium 31mg	2%
Iron 1mg	6%
Potassium 241mg	5%

Avocado-Cheese Bagel

If you are in love with a bagel, you will enjoy making an avocado-cheese bagel recipe.

- Prep Time: 5 minutes
- Cook Time: 0 minutes
- Total Time: 5 minutes
- Serving: 1

<u>Ingredients</u>

- 1 white gluten-free bread, toasted
- 2 tablespoons lactose-free Swiss cheese
- ½ avocado, mashed
- Salt to taste

<u>Instructions</u>

- Open the bagel and coat a half with cheese, avocado (mashed), and salt.
- Cover with the other half. Enjoy!

<u>Cooking Tips:</u>

- You may want to add fresh lemon juice to your avocado for another great taste and avoid turning avocado to brown.

Nutrition Facts	
Servings: 1	
Amount per serving	
Calories	**525**
	% Daily Value*
Total Fat 21.3g	27%
Saturated Fat 4.4g	22%
Cholesterol 3mg	1%
Sodium 896mg	39%
Total Carbohydrate 66.2g	24%
Dietary Fiber 9.3g	33%
Total Sugars 6.3g	
Protein 19.9g	
Vitamin D 0mcg	0%
Calcium 210mg	16%
Iron 5mg	28%
Potassium 572mg	12%

PINEAPPLE-GINSENG OATMEAL

Another great recipe for oatmeal with amazing mix flavors of ginseng and pineapple.

- Prep Time: 5 minutes
- Cook Time: 20 minutes
- Total Time: 25 minutes
- Serving: 4

<u>Ingredients</u>

- 2 cups old-fashioned rolled oats
- 2 cups pineapple chunks
- 1 small piece of ginseng or one teaspoon ginseng powder
- ½ teaspoon salt
- 2 cups unsweetened almond or lactose-free milk
- ½ cups brown sugar
- 2 large organic free-range eggs
- 2 teaspoon vanilla extract

<u>Instructions</u>

- Preheat oven to 375 °F.

- In a medium bowl, mix and whisk oats with ginseng, salt, pineapple, and milk.
- Use a suitable baking pan or sheet. Spread your mix to it and bake for 20 minutes until golden brown.

<u>Cooking Tips:</u>

- You can prepare this breakfast in a large skillet over medium heat until brown.

Nutrition Facts

Servings: 4

Amount per serving	
Calories	**308**
	% Daily Value*
Total Fat 5.6g	7%
Saturated Fat 1.2g	6%
Cholesterol 93mg	31%
Sodium 419mg	18%
Total Carbohydrate 61g	22%
Dietary Fiber 3.8g	14%
Total Sugars 43.9g	
Protein 6.8g	
Vitamin D 9mcg	47%
Calcium 177mg	14%
Iron 2mg	12%
Potassium 250mg	5%

Strawberry Cinnamon Oatmeal

Enjoy tasting a traditional strawberry cinnamon oatmeal that can be prepared in less than 15 minutes.

- Prep Time: 5 minutes
- Cook Time: 15 minutes
- Total Time: 20 minutes
- Serving: 2

<u>Ingredients</u>

- 1 tablespoon extra virgin olive oil
- 1 cup gluten-free ground oats or ready oatmeal
- 2 cups unsweetened almond or lactose-free milk
- ½ teaspoon cinnamon

- 10 strawberries, sliced
- 1 tablespoon brown sugar

Instructions

- Preheat oven to 375 °F.
- In a medium bowl, mix and whisk oats with cinnamon, oil, strawberries, brown sugar, and milk.
- Use a suitable baking pan or sheet. Spread your mix to it and bake for 15 minutes until golden brown.

Cooking Tips:

- You can prepare this breakfast in a large skillet over medium heat for 10-15 minutes until brown.

Nutrition Facts

Servings: 2

Amount per serving

Calories	276
	% Daily Value*
Total Fat 12.5g	16%
Saturated Fat 1.3g	7%
Cholesterol 0mg	0%
Sodium 182mg	8%
Total Carbohydrate 40.6g	15%
Dietary Fiber 6.5g	23%
Total Sugars 17.6g	
Protein 4.8g	
Vitamin D 1mcg	7%
Calcium 323mg	25%
Iron 3mg	15%
Potassium 332mg	7%

APPETIZERS

TURKEY POTPIE SOUP

Great soup with perfect ingredients for people with fructose intolerance.

- Prep Time: 10 minutes
- Cook Time: 35 minutes

- Total Time: 45 minutes
- Serving: 4

<u>Ingredients</u>

- ¼ cup white gluten-free flour
- 16 oz turkey breast, cubed
- 2 cups turkey/chicken stock, divided
- 4 cups lactose-free cow milk
- 1 teaspoon turmeric powder
- 1 celery stalks, chopped in small pieces or half a cup celery juice
- 1 large carrot, cubed 1 inch (~2.54 cm)
- 2 medium potatoes, peeled and cubed 1 inch (~2.54 cm)
- Salt and pepper, to taste

<u>Instructions</u>

1. Mix 1 cup of turkey/chicken broth with flour and whisk well. Set aside.
2. Pour another cup of broth into a large pot. Add turkey, celery, potatoes and turmeric powder inside and boil until vegetables and turkey get soft.
3. Warm milk and add to the mix. Then, add carrots and cook for another 5 minutes. Add salt and pepper to taste.

<u>Cooking Tips:</u>

- You can remove flour from the recipe if you do not have one or do not want a soup with a thick texture.
- You can make this soup with chicken breasts as well.

<u>Fructose Intolerance-related Tips:</u>

- Some references recommend celery juice for people with fructose intolerance instead of cubed celeries. Hence, it is recommended to try celery juice first and have it in your recipe only if you can tolerate it.

Nutrition Facts

Servings: 4

Amount per serving

Calories	326
	% Daily Value*
Total Fat 2.4g	3%
Saturated Fat 0.5g	3%
Cholesterol 54mg	18%
Sodium 1696mg	74%
Total Carbohydrate 42.3g	15%
Dietary Fiber 4.2g	15%
Total Sugars 18.6g	
Protein 30.6g	
Vitamin D 1mcg	6%
Calcium 341mg	26%
Iron 3mg	16%
Potassium 1286mg	27%

POTATO-GINSENG MISO SOUP

A fabulous Miso soup with GI healing ingredients. A great source of required vitamins and minerals for people with fructose intolerance:

- Prep Time: 10 minutes
- Cook Time: 30 minutes
- Total Time: 40 minutes
- Serving: 3-4

<u>Ingredients</u>

- 1 fresh ginseng or ½ tablespoon fresh grated ginseng
- 2 cups sodium-free/low sodium vegetable broth
- 2 tablespoons miso

- 2 medium potatoes, peeled and cubed 1 inch (~2.54 cm)
- ½ cup unsweetened almond milk
- ½ teaspoon salt
- ½ teaspoon garlic powder (optional)

<u>Instructions</u>

1. Boil potatoes in a medium pot until softened.
2. Drain and mash your potatoes.
3. In a medium/large pot, mix broth, ginseng, salt, and garlic powder (optional) and boil over medium heat.
4. Add mashed potatoes to the mix and blend until smoothened.
5. Add warm miso and almond milk. Blend again until smoothened. Then, heat the soup for 5 more minutes over medium heat. Enjoy!

<u>Cooking Tips:</u>

- You can add 1 cup of chicken breast to the recipe if you want to have chicken miso.

<u>Fructose Intolerance-related Tips:</u>

- Do not use garlic powder if you cannot tolerate it.

Nutrition Facts

Servings: 3

Amount per serving

Calories 242

% Daily Value*

Total Fat 11.3g	15%
Saturated Fat 8.9g	45%
Cholesterol 0mg	0%
Sodium 951mg	41%
Total Carbohydrate 28.8g	10%
Dietary Fiber 5g	18%
Total Sugars 4.2g	
Protein 8g	
Vitamin D 0mcg	0%
Calcium 33mg	3%
Iron 2mg	12%
Potassium 857mg	18%

PARSNIP/CARROT POTATO SOUP

The parsnip is a root vegetable from the carrot family. Do not use parsnip if you it irritates your gut. Instead, use carrot in the recipe.

- Prep Time: 10 minutes
- Cook Time: 30 minutes
- Total Time: 40 minutes
- Serving: 4

Ingredients

- ½ cup celery juice
- 4 parsnips or carrots, cubed 1 inch (~2.54 cm)
- 3 cups chicken broth
- 1 tablespoon extra virgin olive oil
- 2 potatoes, skin removed and cubed 1 inch (~2.54 cm)
- 1 teaspoon salt
- 2 tablespoons lactose-free Havarti cheese (optional)
- 1 teaspoon pepper (optional)

Instructions

6. Choose a large pan and cook celery juice and parsnip (carrot) using extra virgin olive oil over medium heat and occasionally mix until semi-soft texture.
7. Warm up the broth and pour it into the pan. Add potato, salt, and pepper (optional) and cook for 20 minutes.
8. Enjoy the soup as it is or blend it for having a puree.
9. Sprinkle lactose-free Havarti cheese on top if you desire.

Cooking Tips:

- You can mix all ingredients at the same time and let it boil for 25-30 minutes.

Fructose Intolerance-related Tips:

- Do not use parsnip if you cannot tolerate it. Instead, use carrots.

Nutrition Facts

Servings: 4

Amount per serving

Calories	**184**
	% Daily Value*
Total Fat 4.9g	6%
Saturated Fat 0.9g	4%
Cholesterol 0mg	0%
Sodium 593mg	26%
Total Carbohydrate 29.7g	11%
Dietary Fiber 6g	21%
Total Sugars 5.1g	
Protein 6.3g	
Vitamin D 0mcg	0%
Calcium 45mg	3%
Iron 1mg	7%
Potassium 864mg	18%

PUMPKIN SOUP

Great semi-classical pumpkin soup can be one of your choices to make every week.

- Prep Time: 15 minutes
- Cook Time: 15 minutes
- Total Time: 30 minutes
- Serving: 4-6

<u>Ingredients</u>

- 2 lbs (~1 kg) pumpkin, skin-removed, seeds-removed, chopped
- 1 large carrot, skin-removed, diced
- 2 large potatoes, skin removed, diced
- 4 cups sodium-free/low sodium chicken broth
- ½ cup lactose-free cow milk
- Salt and pepper, to taste
- 2 chicken bouillon cubes (optional)
- 1 tablespoon garlic powder (optional)

<u>Instructions</u>

1. Mix and boil all ingredients in a large pot over medium heat.
2. Remove from heat. Blend the soup until smooth.
3. Add salt, and pepper to taste

<u>Cooking Tips:</u>

- You can also cook vegetables first in a large skillet by 1 tablespoon extra virgin olive oil over medium heat until semi-soft texture. Then, boil and blend.

Nutrition Facts	
Servings: 6	
Amount per serving	
Calories	**174**
	% Daily Value*
Total Fat 1.5g	2%
Saturated Fat 0.5g	3%
Cholesterol 0mg	0%
Sodium 543mg	24%
Total Carbohydrate 34.3g	12%
Dietary Fiber 7.6g	27%
Total Sugars 8.5g	
Protein 7.8g	
Vitamin D 0mcg	1%
Calcium 86mg	7%
Iron 3mg	17%
Potassium 988mg	21%

STRACCIATELLA SOUP

This delicious Italian soup is entirely in line with patient's tolerance levels with full of healthy ingredients. It can significantly supply your protein.

- Prep Time: 10 minutes
- Cook Time: 15 minutes
- Total Time: 25 minutes
- Serving: 4

Ingredients

- 6 cups low sodium/sodium-free chicken broth
- 2 tablespoons all-purpose gluten-free flour
- 3 large organic free-range eggs
- Salt and pepper, to taste
- 1 tablespoon hard pecorino cheese, grated
- 1 tablespoon hard Parmigiano-Reggiano cheese, grated
- 1 tablespoon fresh parsley (optional)

Instructions

1. In a large pot and over high heat, bring chicken stock to simmer. Add salt and pepper.
2. In a large bowl, whisk eggs, semolina or all-purpose gluten-free flour, Parmigiano-Reggiano, and pecorino cheese altogether.
3. Slowly pour the egg mixture into your pot and simmer well. Let the soup simmer.
4. Serve and garnish it with parsley if you want. Enjoy!

Cooking Tips:

- Most aged cheddar-type cheeses are lactose-free. As such, lactose-intolerant patients can tolerate pecorino and Parmigiano-Reggiano. However, they should be used in moderation.

Fructose Intolerance-related Tips:

- Use pecorino and Parmigiano-Reggiano in moderation if you can tolerate them or simply remove them from the recipe.

Nutrition Facts

Servings: 4

Amount per serving

Calories 164

	% Daily Value*
Total Fat 8.3g	11%
Saturated Fat 3.5g	18%
Cholesterol 147mg	49%
Sodium 1277mg	56%
Total Carbohydrate 5.5g	2%
Dietary Fiber 0.2g	1%
Total Sugars 1.3g	
Protein 15.4g	
Vitamin D 13mcg	66%
Calcium 120mg	9%
Iron 2mg	9%
Potassium 376mg	8%

HAM AND POTATO SOUP

A delicious soup for people with fructose intolerance who love ham.

- Prep Time: 10 minutes
- Cook Time: 20 minutes
- Total Time: 30 minutes
- Serving: 4

Ingredients

- 2 large potatoes, peeled and cubed 1 inch (~2.54 cm)
- 1 cup cooked ham, diced and cubed 1 inch (~2.54 cm)
- 3 cups sodium-free/low sodium chicken broth
- 1 tablespoon extra virgin olive oil
- ¼ cup white gluten-free flour
- ½ cup celery stalk, diced
- 2 cups lactose-free cow milk
- Salt and pepper to taste

Instructions

1. Boil potatoes, celery, ham, and chicken broth in a large pot over medium heat for 15 minutes.
2. In a large pan, pour high-quality extra virgin olive oil and whisk flour over medium heat. Stir consistently until golden brown. Warm milk and add slowly to the flour. Stir continuously for five minutes.
3. Pour the mix into the pot and stir. Add salt and pepper to taste. Enjoy!

Fructose Intolerance-related Tips:

- Avoid using honey ham. Instead, use fat-removed pork tenderloin or chicken breasts.

Nutrition Facts	
Servings: 4	
Amount per serving	
Calories	**316**
	% Daily Value*
Total Fat 9.2g	12%
Saturated Fat 3.1g	15%
Cholesterol 29mg	10%
Sodium 935mg	41%
Total Carbohydrate 43.3g	16%
Dietary Fiber 5.3g	19%
Total Sugars 8.2g	
Protein 16.1g	
Vitamin D 1mcg	3%
Calcium 190mg	15%
Iron 2mg	12%
Potassium 1112mg	24%

CHICKEN NOODLE SOUP

The chicken noodle soup is one of the famed soups all around the world. Enjoy making it in less than 45 minutes!

- Prep Time: 5 minutes
- Cook Time: 40 minutes
- Total Time: 45 minutes
- Serving: 6

<u>Ingredients</u>

- 1 cup gluten-free vermicelli or gluten-free egg noodles or rice noodles
- 8 skin-removed chicken legs
- 1-2 chicken bouillon cube(s), crushed
- 2 cups of water
- 1 tablespoon extra virgin olive oil
- 2 teaspoons salt, to taste
- 2 large carrots, cubed & skin-removed
- ½ cup celery juice
- 6 cups low sodium chicken stock/broth
- 1 teaspoon garlic powder (optional)
- 1 teaspoon ground black pepper, to taste (optional)

- ¼ cup fresh parsley, chopped (optional)

<u>Instructions</u>

1. In a large skillet, heat high-quality olive oil over medium heat and cook celery juice and carrots for 5 minutes.
2. Pour chicken broth into the skillet, add and cook chicken legs.
3. Add crushed bouillons and water to cover all ingredients.
4. When chicken cooked, use a plate to shred it and remove the bone.
5. Bring shredded chickens back to the soup and add gluten-free noodles. Add salt, pepper, and garlic powder (optional). Cover it for 7 minutes. Then, open the lid and stir well.
6. Serve in a bowl and garnish with chopped fresh parsley (optional)

<u>Cooking Tips:</u>

- You can use skin-removed chicken thighs or breasts instead of chicken legs, as well.

<u>Fructose Intolerance-related Tips:</u>

- Do not use garlic powder or parsley if you are experiencing a severe flare-up.

Nutrition Facts	
Servings: 6	
Amount per serving	
Calories	**420**
	% Daily Value*
Total Fat 13.9g	18%
Saturated Fat 3.3g	17%
Cholesterol 120mg	40%
Sodium 1175mg	51%
Total Carbohydrate 28.3g	10%
Dietary Fiber 1.8g	6%
Total Sugars 3.2g	
Protein 41.9g	
Vitamin D 0mcg	0%
Calcium 27mg	2%
Iron 3mg	19%
Potassium 346mg	7%

CREAMY CHICKEN SOUP

A very delicious savory soup specially modified for people with fructose intolerance.

- Prep Time: 5 minutes
- Cook Time: 30 minutes
- Total Time: 35 minutes
- Serving: 4-6

<u>Ingredients</u>

- 1.5 lbs boneless, skin-removed chicken breast
- 1 cup carrots, skin-removed and cubed 1 inch (~2.54 cm)
- 1 medium potato, skin-removed and cubed 1 inch (~2.54 cm)
- 2 tablespoons extra virgin olive oil
- 1 cup low-fat lactose-free cow milk
- 3 cups low-sodium chicken broth
- 1 teaspoon turmeric powder
- Salt and pepper, to taste
- ½ teaspoon dried thyme
- 1-2 tablespoon(s) lemon juice

- 1 teaspoon garlic powder (optional)
- 1 cup mushrooms only if you can tolerate it (optional)
- 1 cup lactose-free cream/sour cream (optional)

Instructions

1. Heat extra virgin olive oil in a large pot and cook chicken over medium heat with turmeric, salt, and pepper until golden brown both sides. Remove chickens.
2. Add carrots, potato, thyme, garlic powder (optional), and mushroom (optional) to the pot. Stir well until half-cooked. Add chicken broth. Then, let it cook for 15-20 minutes.
3. Add warm milk and 1-2 tablespoon(s) lemon juice. Let it simmer for five more minutes. Serve warm and enjoy!

Cooking Tips:

- You can try ½ cup shiitake mushroom if regular mushrooms irritate your gut, or remove mushroom from the recipe.
- You can add lactose-free sour cream on top of the soup if you can tolerate it.

Fructose Intolerance-related Tips:

- Do not use garlic powder if you are experiencing a severe flare-up.

Nutrition Facts	
Servings: 6	
Amount per serving	
Calories	**224**
	% Daily Value*
Total Fat 6.7g	9%
Saturated Fat 1g	5%
Cholesterol 68mg	23%
Sodium 145mg	6%
Total Carbohydrate 10.9g	4%
Dietary Fiber 1.4g	5%
Total Sugars 3.4g	
Protein 29.6g	
Vitamin D 21mcg	106%
Calcium 61mg	5%
Iron 2mg	8%
Potassium 285mg	6%

SEAFOOD CHOWDER SOUP

A must-try recipe if you are in love with seafood!

- Prep Time: 10 minutes
- Cook Time: 25 minutes
- Total Time: 35 minutes
- Serving: 4-6

Ingredients

- 3 potatoes, peeled and cubed 1 inch (~2.54 cm)
- 2 cups of low-sodium vegetable broth or chicken broth
- ¾ cup of lactose-free cow milk
- 4 oz salmon filet, peeled and cubed
- 4 oz codfish filet, peeled and cubed
- 8 raw shrimps, peeled
- 2 tablespoons fresh lemon juice
- 1 bay leaf
- ½ teaspoon grated ginseng
- Salt and pepper to taste

Instructions

1. In a large pot, warm chicken broth and add potatoes, bay leaf, salmon, and cod.
2. Let the soup cook for 15 minutes over medium heat. Stir occasionally. Cover but leave a corner open for the steam to escape.
3. Add warm milk, shrimp, lemon juice, ginseng, sale, and pepper to the soup. Stir for 5-10 minutes. Enjoy!

<u>Cooking Tips:</u>

- You can add ⅓ cup of crab into the soup if you like.
- You can add lactose-free sour cream on top of the soup if you can tolerate it.

Nutrition Facts

Servings: 6

Amount per serving	
Calories	**268**
	% Daily Value*
Total Fat 7.1g	9%
Saturated Fat 1.6g	8%
Cholesterol 134mg	45%
Sodium 285mg	12%
Total Carbohydrate 20.5g	7%
Dietary Fiber 3g	11%
Total Sugars 3.7g	
Protein 31.4g	
Vitamin D 0mcg	1%
Calcium 112mg	9%
Iron 2mg	10%
Potassium 772mg	16%

OATMEAL SOUP

A delicious Mediterranean soup with healthy, rich ingredients for people with fructose intolerance!

- Prep Time: 10 minutes
- Soak Time: 120 minutes
- Cook Time: 40 minutes
- Total Time: 50 (or 170) minutes
- Serving: 6

Ingredients

- 1 cup oatmeal
- 1 tablespoon all-purpose gluten-free flour
- 1.5 cup low-fat lactose-free cow milk
- 1 cup carrot, peeled and cubed 1 inch (~2.54 cm)
- 7 cups low-sodium chicken broth
- 1 tablespoon extra virgin olive oil
- 1 tablespoon fresh lemon, squeezed
- Salt & pepper, to taste
- 1 tablespoon parsley, chopped (optional)

Instructions

1. In a large pot, cook oatmeal and carrots with chicken broth over medium heat for 30 minutes. Add salt and pepper. Stir occasionally.
2. In a medium pan, make a béchamel sauce: heat extra virgin olive oil. Add flour to the oil and stir until golden brown. Slowly add warm milk to the pan and stir perfectly until thickened. If the sauce is very thick, add more milk.
3. Add béchamel sauce to the pot and add lemon juice. Stir well over low heat for 5-10 more minutes.
4. Garnish the top with chopped parsley. Enjoy!

Cooking Tips:

- You may want to add ½ cup skin-removed chicken breast to your soup to make a chicken-oatmeal soup.

Fructose Intolerance-related Tips:

- Do not use pepper and parsley if you are experiencing a severe flare-up.

- If you cannot tolerate tomato, do not use the orange version of this soup explained in the cooking tips section.

Nutrition Facts

Servings: 6

Amount per serving

Calories   **185**

	% Daily Value*
Total Fat 3.7g	5%
Saturated Fat 0.9g	4%
Cholesterol 3mg	1%
Sodium 125mg	5%
Total Carbohydrate 29.8g	11%
Dietary Fiber 5.9g	21%
Total Sugars 4.4g	
Protein 8.5g	
Vitamin D 32mcg	159%
Calcium 89mg	7%
Iron 2mg	9%
Potassium 293mg	6%

LENTIL SOUP

A great healthy and easy to cook middle-eastern soup for people with fructose intolerance.

- Prep Time: 5 minutes
- Cook Time: 45 minutes
- Total Time: 50 minutes
- Serving: 4

<u>Ingredients</u>

- ¾ cup green lentils, washed
- 3 cups low-sodium chicken broth or water
- 1 tablespoon extra virgin olive oil
- ½ tablespoon salt, to taste
- ½ tablespoon turmeric powder
- 1 teaspoon cinnamon powder
- ½ teaspoon pepper (optional)
- 1 teaspoon garlic powder (optional)

- 1 teaspoon Angelica powder (optional)

<u>Instructions</u>

1. Choose a large pot and put all ingredients, except Angelica and cinnamon powder into it. Add water or chicken broth and let it boil over high heat.
2. Cover but stir occasionally. Let the lentils cook for 40 minutes over low/medium heat.
3. Add angelical and cinnamon powders. Enjoy!

<u>Cooking Tips:</u>

- You may want to add ½ cup skin-removed chicken breast to your recipe to make a chicken-lentil soup.
- You can blend the soup to have a smooth texture.

<u>Fructose Intolerance-related Tips:</u>

- Do not use garlic powder if you are experiencing a severe flare-up.
- Use lentil in moderation and cook this recipe only during remissions. It can cause bloating in some patients. Avoid using this soup when you are experiencing a flare-up. Alternatively, you can remove lentils and consume the clear broth.

Nutrition Facts	
Servings: 4	
Amount per serving	
Calories	**171**
	% Daily Value*
Total Fat 4g	5%
Saturated Fat 0.6g	3%
Cholesterol 0mg	0%
Sodium 927mg	40%
Total Carbohydrate 22.9g	8%
Dietary Fiber 11.2g	40%
Total Sugars 0.8g	
Protein 10.9g	
Vitamin D 0mcg	0%
Calcium 22mg	2%
Iron 3mg	19%
Potassium 365mg	8%

HOMEMADE VEGETABLE BROTH

It is an excellent idea for people living with fructose intolerance to make their homemade vegetable broth instead of purchasing it from the stores. Many vegetable products are high in sodium and are mixed vegetables that cannot be well-tolerated by fructose intolerance patients.

- Prep Time: 10 minutes
- Cook Time: 45 minutes
- Total Time: 55 minutes
- Serving: 4-6

<u>Ingredients</u>

- 4 cups celery, chopped or 1.5 cup of celery juice
- 4 cups carrot, skin-removed and cubed
- 4 cups of water
- 2 tablespoons fresh lemon juice
- 2 tablespoons extra virgin olive oil
- ½ tablespoon turmeric powder
- 1 bay leaf
- ½ tablespoon salt, to taste
- 1 tablespoon fresh parsley, chopped (optional)

- ½ teaspoon pepper (optional)
- 1 teaspoon garlic powder (optional)

Instructions

1. Choose a large pan and cook vegetables with extra virgin olive oil, turmeric powder, salt, and pepper over medium heat until golden brown.
2. Put ingredients in the pan into a large pot, add water, lemon juice, bay leaf, garlic powder (optional), and chopped fresh parsley (optional). Thoroughly boil over low heat until all ingredients get soft.
3. Clear the broth by a colander. Serve immediately or pour and store in a suitable bottle for further use.

Cooking Tips:

- You can blend all ingredients to have a smoothened soup instead of broth.

Fructose Intolerance-related Tips:

- Do not use pepper, garlic powder, and fresh parsley if you are experiencing a severe flare-up.

Nutrition Facts	
Servings: 4	
Amount per serving	
Calories	**127**
	% Daily Value*
Total Fat 7.4g	9%
Saturated Fat 1.1g	6%
Cholesterol 0mg	0%
Sodium 1038mg	45%
Total Carbohydrate 14.9g	5%
Dietary Fiber 4.7g	17%
Total Sugars 7g	
Protein 1.8g	
Vitamin D 0mcg	0%
Calcium 90mg	7%
Iron 1mg	6%
Potassium 650mg	14%

HOMEMADE BEEF BROTH

An excellent idea for people living with fructose intolerance to make their homemade beef broth instead of purchasing it from the stores. Many vegetable products are high in sodium and fat that are not good for people with fructose intolerance. Beef broth is an excellent option for people with fructose intolerance to consume when they are experiencing a flare-up.

- Prep Time: 10 minutes
- Cook Time: 60 minutes
- Total Time: 70 minutes
- Serving: 4-6

Ingredients

- 6 lbs organic grass-fed beef bones
- 2 celery stalks, chopped, or 1 cup of celery juice
- 3 carrots, chopped
- 3 bay leaves
- 1 teaspoon turmeric
- 1 tablespoon extra virgin olive oil
- 1 teaspoon dried thyme
- 2 tablespoons salt
- 1 teaspoon black pepper (optional)
- 1 teaspoon garlic powder (optional)

Instructions

1. Preheat oven to 400 °F.
2. Roast your bones, celery, carrots with extra virgin olive oil in the oven for 40 minutes.

3. At the same time, boil water and add bay leaves, turmeric, thyme, salt, pepper, and garlic powder (optional) to it.
4. Add the roasted bones and vegetables to the water. Water should be enough to cover all ingredients.
5. Lid ajar and simmer all mix over slow heat for 20 minutes.
6. Remove all bones.
7. Clear the broth by a colander. Serve immediately or pour and store in a suitable bottle or jar for further use.

<u>Cooking Tips:</u>

- You can blend all ingredients to have a smoothened soup instead of broth, especially if you cooked meat pieces with bones.

<u>Fructose Intolerance-related Tips:</u>

- Do not use pepper and garlic powder if you are experiencing a flare-up.

Nutrition Facts

Servings: 4

Amount per serving	
Calories	**122**
	% Daily Value*
Total Fat 5.2g	7%
Saturated Fat 2.1g	10%
Cholesterol 15mg	5%
Sodium 460mg	20%
Total Carbohydrate 14g	5%
Dietary Fiber 3.3g	12%
Total Sugars 4g	
Protein 9.6g	
Vitamin D 0mcg	0%
Calcium 37mg	3%
Iron 1mg	7%
Potassium 433mg	9%

RUSSIAN CHICKEN SOUP

A great, easy to cook Russian soup for cold winters. Great ingredients for people with fructose intolerance!

- Prep Time: 10 minutes
- Cook Time: 30 minutes
- Total Time: 40 minutes
- Serving: 6

Ingredients

- 3 lbs organic, grass-fed chicken breasts, cubed 1 inch (~2.54 cm)
- ¾ cup gluten-free pasta
- 4 cups low-sodium chicken or vegetable broth, or water
- 1 tablespoon extra virgin olive oil
- 1 carrot, skin-removed and cubed 1 inch (~2.54 cm)
- 4 medium potatoes, cubed & peeled 1 inch (~2.54 cm)
- 2 tablespoons fresh lemon juice
- 1 bay leaf
- Salt and pepper, to taste
- 1 teaspoon garlic powder (optional)

Instructions

1. Put all ingredients (except lemon juice and carrot) in a large pot and let it simmer over medium heat for 25 minutes.
2. Add carrots and lemon juice to the soup. Cook it for five more minutes. Then, adjust salt and pepper as desired.
3. Enjoy!

Cooking Tips:

- You can also fry chicken and carrot in a pan by one tablespoon of extra virgin olive oil and 1-teaspoon turmeric powder until golden brown. Then add chicken and carrot to the soup.

<u>Fructose Intolerance-related Tips:</u>

- Do not use pepper and garlic powder if you are experiencing a flare-up.

Nutrition Facts

Servings: 6

Amount per serving	
Calories	**276**
	% Daily Value*
Total Fat 5g	6%
Saturated Fat 1.1g	5%
Cholesterol 66mg	22%
Sodium 70mg	3%
Total Carbohydrate 32.4g	12%
Dietary Fiber 3.8g	13%
Total Sugars 2.2g	
Protein 24.6g	
Vitamin D 0mcg	0%
Calcium 35mg	3%
Iron 2mg	11%
Potassium 779mg	17%

SALMON BRUSCHETTA

Experience great tastes of salmon, bread, and cheese!

- Prep Time: 10 minutes
- Cook Time: 30 minutes
- Total Time: 40 minutes
- Serving: 4

<u>Ingredients</u>

- ½ cup smoked salmon, thinly sliced
- 8 gluten-free bread/baguette slices
- ½ cup low-fat lactose-free cheese such as Swiss
- 1 tablespoon grated horseradish

- 1 tablespoon fresh lemon juice
- 1 tablespoon extra virgin olive oil
- 1 cup Persian cucumbers, peeled & chopped
- 1 teaspoon lemon zest

Instructions

1. Cut your baguette to have 1-inch (~2.54 cm) pieces. Then, toast your baguette pieces.
2. Mix cheese, horseradish, olive oil, lemon juice, and zest in a bowl. Grate cucumbers in it.
3. Spread your mix on toast slices and put smoked salmon on top. Enjoy!

Nutrition Facts

Servings: 4

Amount per serving

Calories	224
	% Daily Value*
Total Fat 14.8g	19%
Saturated Fat 7.2g	36%
Cholesterol 36mg	12%
Sodium 388mg	17%
Total Carbohydrate 14.9g	5%
Dietary Fiber 0.8g	3%
Total Sugars 1.1g	
Protein 8.2g	
Vitamin D 0mcg	0%
Calcium 38mg	3%
Iron 1mg	8%
Potassium 110mg	2%

Guacamole-Like Appetizer

A modified guacamole recipe for people with fructose intolerance.

- Prep Time: 5 minutes
- Cook Time: 0 minutes
- Total Time: 5 minutes
- Serving: 4-6

Ingredients

- 4 avocados, peeled
- ½ tablespoon extra virgin olive oil
- ¼ cup chopped fresh cilantro
- 2 tablespoons fresh lime juice
- 1 teaspoon fresh lemon juice
- ½ teaspoon salt

Instructions

1- In a large bowl, mash avocados.
2- Add extra virgin olive oil and other ingredients into it.
3- Enjoy!

Cooking Tips:

- You can serve guacamole with gluten-free tacos.
- If you can tolerate tomatoes and onions (in small amounts), cube, and add them into your guacamole.

Fructose Intolerance-related Tips:

- Do not take taco chips with gluten.
- Always consume avocado in moderation.

Nutrition Facts

Servings: 6

Amount per serving	
Calories	**422**
	% Daily Value*
Total Fat 40.4g	52%
Saturated Fat 8.4g	42%
Cholesterol 0mg	0%
Sodium 207mg	9%
Total Carbohydrate 18g	7%
Dietary Fiber 13.5g	48%
Total Sugars 1.2g	
Protein 3.9g	
Vitamin D 0mcg	0%
Calcium 26mg	2%
Iron 1mg	7%
Potassium 988mg	21%

HOMEMADE LEBANESE HUMMUS

A healthy and tasty middle-eastern appetizer. An excellent option for vegetarians and people with fructose intolerance in remission.

- Prep Time: 5 minutes
- Cook Time: 60 minutes
- Total Time: 65 minutes
- Serving: 4

<u>Ingredients</u>

- ¼ lb dried chickpeas (soaked in water for one night)
- 1½ tablespoons tahini
- 1 tablespoon lemon juice
- 2 tablespoons extra virgin olive oil, divided
- ¼ teaspoon cumin
- ½ teaspoon salt
- 1 tablespoon water
- 1 teaspoon baking soda (optional)
- 1 teaspoon paprika powder (optional)
- ½ teaspoon garlic powder (optional)

<u>Instructions</u>

1- First, the you need to soak the chickpeas overnight in water and optionally add baking soda to the water.
2- Cook your chickpeas in a large pot with water over medium heat for about 1 hour. Check if chickpeas cooked well by crushing one of them with a fork in your hand.
3- When chickpeas cooked, drain them and put them in a blender.

4- Add 1 tablespoon of extra virgin olive oil, lemon juice, tahini, cumin powder, salt, and garlic powder (optional) to the blender. Blend until your hummus gets a soft, creamy texture equally.

5- Sprinkle with 1 tablespoon extra virgin olive oil or paprika powder (optional).

6- Serve immediately or fridge it.

Cooking Tips:

- Hummus is well-matched with white gluten-free pita bread.
- You can serve hummus, hot or cold.

Fructose Intolerance-related Tips:

- Do not use paprika and garlic powders in hummus if you are experiencing a severe flare-up.
- Always eat hummus in moderation. During a flare-up, it is better not to make this recipe or make and consume in a small amount.

Nutrition Facts	
Servings: 4	
Amount per serving	
Calories	**198**
	% Daily Value*
Total Fat 11.8g	15%
Saturated Fat 1.6g	8%
Cholesterol 0mg	0%
Sodium 305mg	13%
Total Carbohydrate 18.5g	7%
Dietary Fiber 5.5g	20%
Total Sugars 3.1g	
Protein 6.5g	
Vitamin D 0mcg	0%
Calcium 56mg	4%
Iron 2mg	13%
Potassium 279mg	6%

CRAB DIP WITH GLUTEN-FREE WONTON CHIPS

A great, easy-to-make appetizer with crabs in wonton wrappers!

- Prep Time: 5 minutes
- Cook Time: 30 minutes
- Total Time: 35 minutes
- Serving: 6

<u>Ingredients</u>

- 1 package gluten-free wonton wrappers
- 1 teaspoon extra virgin olive oil
- 1 can crab meat, chopped
- ½ cup organic mayonnaise
- 1 tablespoon soy sauce (optional)
- ½ cup lactose-free cheese
- ½ teaspoon lemon juice
- 1 scallion, chopped
- 1 tablespoon brown sugar
- 1 teaspoon salt, divided
- ½ teaspoon garlic powder (optional)
- ½ teaspoon black pepper (optional)

<u>Instructions</u>

1- Preheat oven to 400 °F.
2- Mix all ingredients into a large mixing bowl. Stir well.
3- In a baking dish, pour all the mix and bake for 30 minutes until you see edge bubbles.
4- Diagonally cut wonton wrappers in half and make triangles. Alternatively, you can make wonton cups.
5- Pour the cups with your mix.

6- Spray extra virgin olive oil on a baking sheet. Put triangles on it and spray olive oil on wontons as well. Add salt as desired. Let the wontons bake for 7 minutes until golden brown.

7- Remove from the oven. Serve and Enjoy!

Cooking Tips:

- You need to watch wontons while baking carefully. They can be burnt fast.

Fructose Intolerance-related Tips:

- Do not use pepper and garlic powders if you are experiencing a severe flare-up.
- When experiencing a flare-up, boil scallion first and then add it to the mix.
- Use soy sauce only if you can tolerate it.

Nutrition Facts

Servings: 6

Amount per serving

Calories	223
	% Daily Value*
Total Fat 14.5g	19%
Saturated Fat 5.4g	27%
Cholesterol 46mg	15%
Sodium 881mg	38%
Total Carbohydrate 16.2g	6%
Dietary Fiber 0.3g	1%
Total Sugars 4.3g	
Protein 7.5g	
Vitamin D 0mcg	0%
Calcium 48mg	4%
Iron 1mg	6%
Potassium 129mg	3%

SHRIMP SALAD

Are you looking for a delicious salad with shrimp? You can follow this recipe to have one!

- Prep Time: 5 minutes

- Cook Time: 15 minutes
- Total Time: 20 minutes
- Serving: 2-4

<u>Ingredients</u>

- 1 lb shrimp, peeled
- ¼ cup celery juice
- 1 tablespoon extra virgin olive oil
- 1 tablespoon fresh lemon juice
- 1 teaspoon Dijon mustard
- ½ teaspoon turmeric powder
- Salt and pepper, to taste
- 2 tablespoons organic low-fat mayonnaise (optional)

<u>Instructions</u>

1. Cook shrimps by extra virgin olive oil and turmeric in a medium pan over medium heat.
2. In a large bowl, mix all lemon juice, celery juice, Dijon mustard, salt, pepper, and mayonnaise (optional).
3. Add cooked shrimp to the bowl and combine.
4. Serve and enjoy!

<u>Cooking Tips:</u>

- You can prepare your shrimps in the oven as well. Just preheat oven to 375 °F. Choose a cooking sheet and spray olive oil on it. Put shrimp on your cooking sheet and let it cook until golden brown (around 10 minutes).

<u>Fructose Intolerance-related Tips:</u>

- Do not use pepper and lots of mayonnaise if you are experiencing a flare-up.

Nutrition Facts	
Servings: 4	
Amount per serving	
Calories	**197**
	% Daily Value*
Total Fat 8g	10%
Saturated Fat 1.5g	7%
Cholesterol 241mg	80%
Sodium 347mg	15%
Total Carbohydrate 3.9g	1%
Dietary Fiber 0.2g	1%
Total Sugars 0.6g	
Protein 26g	
Vitamin D 0mcg	0%
Calcium 107mg	8%
Iron 1mg	3%
Potassium 217mg	5%

ZUCCHINI SALAD (SPIRALIZED)

A great summer salad based on a zucchini. Zucchini salad is a healthy choice for people with fructose intolerance.

- Prep Time: 30 minutes
- Total Time: 30 minutes
- Serving: 2-4

Ingredients

- 2 zucchinis, chopped
- ¼ cup low-fat/fat-free lactose-free aged cheddar
- 1 tablespoon extra virgin olive oil
- 2 tablespoons fresh lemon juice
- 1 tablespoon parsley, chopped (optional)
- Salt and pepper, to taste

Instructions

1. Make spiral zucchinis or cut them thin and lengthwise
2. In a large bowl, mix zucchinis and all other ingredients.
3. For better taste, let it rest for 15 minutes. Enjoy!

<u>Cooking Tips:</u>

- You can use vegetable peelers if you do not have a spiralizer.

<u>Fructose Intolerance-related Tips:</u>

- Do not use pepper if you are experiencing a severe flare-up.
- Check if you can tolerate fresh parsley well or not. If you cannot tolerate, remove it from the recipe.

Nutrition Facts

Servings: 4

Amount per serving

Calories	65
	% Daily Value*
Total Fat 3.7g	5%
Saturated Fat 0.6g	3%
Cholesterol 2mg	1%
Sodium 141mg	6%
Total Carbohydrate 3.9g	1%
Dietary Fiber 1.1g	4%
Total Sugars 1.9g	
Protein 4.8g	
Vitamin D 0mcg	0%
Calcium 65mg	5%
Iron 0mg	2%
Potassium 266mg	6%

OLIVIER SALAD (CHICKEN, POTATO & EGG SALAD)

A traditional well-known Russian salad with great ingredients for people with fructose intolerance. For having a better taste, you can refrigerate it for 30 minutes.

- Prep Time: 15 minutes
- Cook Time: 45 minutes
- Total Time: 60 minutes
- Serving: 6

<u>Ingredients</u>

- 4 potatoes, skin removed and chopped

- 2 cups chicken breasts, shredded
- 2 organic, free-range eggs
- 2 medium carrots
- 1 dill pickles, cubed
- 2 tablespoons extra virgin olive oil
- 2 tablespoons fresh lemon juice
- 1 cup organic low-fat mayonnaise
- Salt and pepper, to taste

Instructions

1. Cook eggs, potatoes, and carrots in a large pot over medium/high heat. Use enough water to cover all ingredients.
2. Mash potatoes and eggs. Cube carrots and pickles (0.3-inch size).
3. In a large bowl, mix all ingredients well.
4. Refrigerate it for 10-15 minutes. Enjoy!

Cooking Tips:

- You can cube your potatoes and eggs similar to carrots, instead of mashing them.

Fructose Intolerance-related Tips:

- Do not use too much pepper and mayonnaise if you are experiencing a flare-up.
- Avoid using dill pickles if you cannot tolerate it. Some recommends not to use sweet pickles at all.
- Always use mayo in moderation. If you cannot tolerate, use plain lactose-free yogurt instead.

Nutrition Facts	
Servings: 6	
Amount per serving	
Calories	**300**
	% Daily Value*
Total Fat 10.2g	13%
Saturated Fat 2.2g	11%
Cholesterol 111mg	37%
Sodium 931mg	40%
Total Carbohydrate 28.6g	10%
Dietary Fiber 4.4g	16%
Total Sugars 5.5g	
Protein 23.8g	
Vitamin D 5mcg	26%
Calcium 40mg	3%
Iron 2mg	11%
Potassium 758mg	16%

PINEAPPLE-PAPAYA SALAD

A simple great fruit salad for everyone!

- Prep Time: 10 minutes
- Total Time: 10 minutes
- Serving: 4-6

Ingredients

- 1 cooked pineapple, chopped
- 1 papaya, peeled and chopped
- ¼ cup brown sugar
- 3 tablespoons fresh lemon juice
- ¼ cup fresh mint leaves, chopped (optional)

Instructions

1. Add all your ingredients in a large bowl and mix well.
2. Serve cold. Enjoy!

Fructose Intolerance-related Tips:

- Check if you can tolerate fresh mint leaves or not. Remove from ingredients if you cannot tolerate it.

Nutrition Facts	
Servings: 4	
Amount per serving	
Calories	**278**
	% Daily Value*
Total Fat 0.8g	1%
Saturated Fat 0.1g	1%
Cholesterol 0mg	0%
Sodium 13mg	1%
Total Carbohydrate 73.2g	27%
Dietary Fiber 10.4g	37%
Total Sugars 56.5g	
Protein 1.6g	
Vitamin D 0mcg	0%
Calcium 33mg	3%
Iron 1mg	7%
Potassium 529mg	11%

CARROT & PINEAPPLE SALAD

A colorful salad with amazing fruits and vegetables inside!

- Prep Time: 10 minutes
- Total Time: 10 minutes
- Serving: 4-6

Ingredients

- 2 medium carrots, peeled and cubed 1 inch (~2.54 cm)
- 4 pineapple slices, cubed 1 inch (~2.54 cm)
- 3 tablespoons fresh orange juice
- 2 tablespoons fresh lime juice
- 1 tablespoon extra virgin olive oil
- Salt and pepper, to taste
- ¼ cup fresh mint leaves, chopped (optional)

Instructions

1. In a large bowl, mix well all ingredients.
2. Serve cold. Enjoy!

Cooking Tips:

- You can add two tablespoons of balsamic vinegar if your gut can tolerate it.

<u>Fructose Intolerance-related Tips:</u>

- Check if you can tolerate fresh mint leaves or not. Remove from ingredients if you cannot tolerate it.
- Do not use pepper if you are experiencing a severe flare-up.

Nutrition Facts

Servings: 4

Amount per serving

Calories	129
	% Daily Value*
Total Fat 3.8g	5%
Saturated Fat 0.5g	3%
Cholesterol 0mg	0%
Sodium 109mg	5%
Total Carbohydrate 24.1g	9%
Dietary Fiber 4.4g	16%
Total Sugars 17.5g	
Protein 2.4g	
Vitamin D 0mcg	0%
Calcium 30mg	2%
Iron 1mg	8%
Potassium 539mg	11%

BUTTER LETTUCE SALAD WITH VINAIGRETTE

A light and delicious salad for people with fructose intolerance who can tolerate butter lettuce with a delicious dressing.

- Prep Time: 15 minutes
- Total Time: 15 minutes
- Serving: 4-6

<u>Ingredients</u>

- 2 medium butter lettuces, cut into small pieces (also called Bibb, Boston or living lettuce)
- 1 tablespoon brown sugar

- 1 teaspoon Dijon mustard
- 2 tablespoons fresh lemon juice
- 2 tablespoons fresh lime juice
- 2 tablespoons extra virgin olive oil
- Salt and pepper to taste

Instructions

1. Wash butter lettuce thoroughly and cut into small pieces
2. In a large bowl, mix well all ingredients.
3. Serve cold. Enjoy!

Cooking Tips:

- You can add two peeled Persian cucumbers to have a garden-like salad!
- You can add one tablespoon of balsamic vinegar if your gut can tolerate it.

Fructose Intolerance-related Tips:

- Butter lettuce, also called Bibb, living or Boston lettuce, is a type of lettuce that can be digested easier than other types of lettuce. Hence, it might be an option for people with fructose intolerance to try. Try butter lettuce and check if you can tolerate it or not. Many of fructose intolerance patients can enjoy a garden salad with butter lettuce during remissions. Avoid making this recipe if you found butter lettuce gut-irritative.
- Do not use pepper if you are experiencing a severe flare-up.

CARROT-AVOCADO SALAD

An epic salad recipe with avocado and tasty dressing. A great salad option for people with fructose intolerance!

- Prep Time: 20 minutes
- Cook Time: 30 minutes
- Total Time: 50 minutes
- Serving: 4-6

Ingredients

- 1 large avocado
- 2 carrots, peeled and diced 1-inch (~2.54 cm)
- 2 tablespoons extra virgin olive oil
- 1 tablespoon fresh lemon juice
- Salt and pepper, to taste
- ⅓ cup green onion, chopped (optional)
- ¼ cup fresh mint leaves, chopped (optional)

Instructions

1. Peel-off carrots.
2. In a small pot, cook carrots in boiling water over medium heat.

3. Cube carrots and avocados. In a medium bowl, mix other ingredients and then add carrot and avocado.
4. Mix well. Enjoy!

<u>Cooking Tips:</u>

- You can cook carrots in a small pan with one tablespoon of extra virgin olive oil and ½ teaspoon of turmeric powder over medium heat as well.

<u>Fructose Intolerance-related Tips:</u>

- Make sure your gut can tolerate green onion before using it.
- Do not use pepper, green onion, and fresh mint if you are experiencing a flare-up.

Nutrition Facts

Servings: 4

Amount per serving

Calories **179**

	% Daily Value*
Total Fat 16.9g	22%
Saturated Fat 3.1g	15%
Cholesterol 0mg	0%
Sodium 26mg	1%
Total Carbohydrate 8g	3%
Dietary Fiber 4.4g	16%
Total Sugars 2g	
Protein 1.4g	
Vitamin D 0mcg	0%
Calcium 22mg	2%
Iron 1mg	3%
Potassium 369mg	8%

CLASSIC TUNA PASTA SALAD

Classic tuna with pasta is an excellent choice as your salad. You can have it for lunch or dinner as well.

- Prep Time: 15 minutes
- Cook Time: 15 minutes
- Total Time: 30 minutes

- Serving: 4

<u>Ingredients</u>

- 1½ cups gluten-free pasta
- 1 celery stalk, chopped, or ½ cup celery juice
- 1 can tuna in water
- ½ cup organic low-fat mayonnaise
- 2 tablespoons white vinegar
- Salt and pepper, to taste

<u>Instructions</u>

1. Cook pasta according to its package instruction.
2. Drain pasta and place it in a large bowl.
3. Add celery, tuna, and all other ingredients to the pasta bowl. Mix well.
4. It is better to let it cool in the fridge for 30 minutes. Enjoy!

<u>Cooking Tips:</u>

- Instead of white vinegar, you can use one tablespoon of fresh lemon juice.

<u>Fructose Intolerance-related Tips:</u>

- Do not use pepper if you are experiencing a flare-up.

Nutrition Facts

Servings: 4

Amount per serving

Calories   **105**

	% Daily Value*
Total Fat 3g	4%
Saturated Fat 0.7g	3%
Cholesterol 25mg	8%
Sodium 526mg	23%
Total Carbohydrate 8.9g	3%
Dietary Fiber 1.4g	5%
Total Sugars 4.9g	
Protein 10.4g	
Vitamin D 0mcg	0%
Calcium 13mg	1%
Iron 1mg	3%
Potassium 159mg	3%

Salmon Ceviche

This salad is full of omega-3 with a fabulous dressing. Enjoy this dairy-free, egg-free, nut-free, and gluten-free recipe.

- Prep Time: 15 minutes
- Rest Time: 15 minutes
- Total Time: 30 minutes
- Serving: 4

Ingredients

- 1 lb salmon, skin removed and cubed
- 1 cup Persian cucumber, cubed 1cm
- ½ cup green onion, chopped well
- 1 tablespoon fresh lemon juice
- 1 tablespoon fresh lime juice
- 1 tablespoon grated fresh ginseng
- Salt and pepper, to taste
- 1 teaspoon dried oregano (optional)

Instructions

1. In a large bowl, mix salmon, cucumber, green onion, ginseng, and oregano.
2. In a small cup/bowl, whisk lime & lemon juice, salt, and pepper and pour it into the large bowl.
3. Mix all well. Serve cold. Enjoy!

<u>Cooking Tips:</u>

- You can add ½ teaspoon freshly grated turmeric if you want to enjoy its anti-inflammatory properties.

<u>Fructose Intolerance-related Tips:</u>

- Make sure your gut can tolerate green onion and oregano before using them.
- Do not use pepper if you are experiencing a flare-up.

Nutrition Facts

Servings: 4

Amount per serving

Calories	**167**
	% Daily Value*
Total Fat 7.1g	9%
Saturated Fat 1.1g	5%
Cholesterol 50mg	17%
Sodium 53mg	2%
Total Carbohydrate 3.9g	1%
Dietary Fiber 1.1g	4%
Total Sugars 0.6g	
Protein 22.4g	
Vitamin D 0mcg	0%
Calcium 52mg	4%
Iron 1mg	6%
Potassium 506mg	11%

CHICKEN SALAD

Enjoy making a rich salad with chicken and mustard. Excellent source of protein for people with fructose intolerance.

- Prep Time: 25 minutes
- Total Time: 25 minutes

- Serving: 4-6

Ingredients

- 1 lb chicken breasts, skinless and boneless
- 1 avocado, chopped
- 3 tablespoons brown sugar
- 2 cups butter lettuce, chopped
- 3 tablespoons apple cider vinegar (optional)
- 2 tablespoons Dijon mustard
- 1 tablespoon lactose-free aged cheddar
- 2 tablespoons extra virgin olive oil
- Salt and pepper, to taste
- ½ teaspoon garlic powder (optional)
- 1 tablespoon green onion, chopped (optional)

Instructions

1. In a large pan, cook chickens with two tablespoons of extra virgin olive oil over medium heat until getting close to a golden brown. Remove from pan and cut into 1-inch (~2.54 cm) cubes.
2. In a large bowl, whisk brown sugar, mustard, vinegar, garlic powder (optional), green onion (optional), cheese, salt, and pepper.
3. In another large bowl, cut butter lettuce into small pieces. Add cubed chickens and pour the sauce on top. Serve and enjoy!

Cooking Tips:

- You can boil chickens in a pot over medium heat (recommended for flare-up times).

Fructose Intolerance-related Tips:

- Make sure your gut can tolerate butter lettuce and green onion before using it.
- Do not use pepper and garlic powder if you are experiencing a flare-up.
- Do not consume apple cider vinegar if you cannot tolerate it.

Nutrition Facts

Servings: 6

Amount per serving

Calories	310
	% Daily Value*
Total Fat 17.1g	22%
Saturated Fat 3.6g	18%
Cholesterol 68mg	23%
Sodium 152mg	7%
Total Carbohydrate 16.5g	6%
Dietary Fiber 2.8g	10%
Total Sugars 12.3g	
Protein 23.6g	
Vitamin D 0mcg	0%
Calcium 29mg	2%
Iron 3mg	15%
Potassium 444mg	9%

MAIN COURSES

MEDITERRANEAN CHICKEN - ZUCCHINI STEW

Chicken–Zucchini stew is one of the delicious Mediterranean stews, which typically serves with steamed white rice. Turmeric, zucchini, and white rice are great for people with fructose intolerance, and most can well-tolerate them.

- Prep Time: 10 minutes
- Cook Time: 50 minutes
- Total Time: 60 minutes
- Serving: 4

<u>Ingredients</u>

- 4 Fresh zucchinis, lengthwise-cut with no skin

- 6 Skin-removed chicken legs
- 4 tablespoons extra virgin olive oil
- 1.5 teaspoon turmeric
- ½ teaspoon black pepper
- 1½ teaspoons salt
- 3 tablespoons lemon juice or 1 lime
- 2½ cups water

<u>Preparation</u>

1. Fry, both sides of skinless zucchinis with two tablespoons of extra virgin olive oil in a sauté pan until golden brown.
2. In another pan, fry your chicken legs with the rest of extra virgin olive oil, salt, pepper, and turmeric until golden brown.
3. Add your chicken legs to the boiling water. Turn the heat to medium. Let it simmer for 20 minutes. If your sauce gets thick, add more water to your stew.
4. After 25 minutes, add your zucchinis and your lemon juice to the stew and let it cook for another 5 minutes. After three minutes, taste your stew and correct your seasonings. Do not add more black peppers.
5. Enjoy this meal with steamed white rice!

<u>Cooking Tips:</u>

- To reach a faster cooking time, you can add all the ingredients into the boiling water and let the stew cook for 40 minutes on high heat.

Nutrition Facts

Servings: 4

Amount per serving

Calories   **352**

	% Daily Value*
Total Fat 22.6g	29%
Saturated Fat 4.4g	22%
Cholesterol 89mg	30%
Sodium 1001mg	44%
Total Carbohydrate 10.5g	4%
Dietary Fiber 3.1g	11%
Total Sugars 5.6g	
Protein 28.9g	
Vitamin D 0mcg	0%
Calcium 55mg	4%
Iron 3mg	16%
Potassium 945mg	20%

Lactose-Free Chicken Fettuccine Alfredo

Do you love to have a creamy-but-healthy Fettuccine Alfredo? You can use this recipe to have a delicious Italian main course. This meal has chicken/vegetable stock, turmeric, ginseng, and lemon that are great for people with fructose intolerance.

- Prep Time: 15 minutes
- Cook Time: 30 minutes
- Total Time: 45 minutes
- Serving: 4

<u>Ingredients</u>

- 4 boneless, skinless chicken breasts, about 0.8 inches (~2 cm) thick
- ¾ lb uncooked gluten-free fettuccine/pasta (~340 g)
- 3 tablespoons gluten-free flour
- 10 oz lactose-free milk (~300 ml)
- ½ cup unsalted organic chicken stock or vegetable stock (~120 ml)
- 1 tablespoon fresh lemon juice
- 3½ teaspoons Himalayan salt, divided

- 2 teaspoons black pepper, divided
- 1 teaspoon turmeric
- 1 teaspoon ginseng powder
- 3 tablespoons extra virgin olive oil, divided
- 1 teaspoon garlic powder (optional)
- Fresh parsley, minced (optional)

<u>Preparation</u>

1. Heat a tablespoon of extra virgin olive oil in a pan. Add your chicken breast with one tablespoon of salt, one tablespoon of pepper and turmeric and let it cook for 5 minutes until golden brown both sides.
2. Boil the water in a large pot over high heat. Add one tablespoon of high-quality extra virgin olive oil and one tablespoon of salt to the water. Then, add your fettuccine in the boiling water.
3. Cook fettuccine according to its package instructions. Drain and return to the pot.
4. In another pan, put one tablespoon of extra virgin olive oil on medium heat. When heated, add your flour slowly and whisk until golden brown.
5. Heat your lactose-free milk in the microwave, add it slowly to your flour, and whisk for 3 minutes. Add lemon juice, ginseng powder, garlic powder (optional), one tablespoon of pepper, and one tablespoon of salt to make an excellent béchamel sauce.
6. Add chicken/vegetable stock to the béchamel sauce, frequently stir for 10 minutes until thickened.
7. Slice or cube chicken. Add the béchamel sauce to your fettuccine pot and toss perfectly.
8. Garnish the top with minced parsley and enjoy!

<u>Fructose Intolerance-related Tips:</u>

- Do not use garlic powder or parsley if you cannot tolerate it.
- Make sure that your chickens are skinless.

Nutrition Facts
Servings: 4

Amount per serving
Calories 626

	% Daily Value*
Total Fat 23.2g	30%
Saturated Fat 5.1g	25%
Cholesterol 170mg	57%
Sodium 2433mg	106%
Total Carbohydrate 51g	19%
Dietary Fiber 3.6g	13%
Total Sugars 1.3g	
Protein 50.5g	
Vitamin D 0mcg	0%
Calcium 52mg	4%
Iron 4mg	20%
Potassium 387mg	8%

CHICKEN WITH MASHED POTATOES

For those who want a very simple but delicious main course. Cooked baby carrot can be used as a well-matched garnish.

- Prep Time: 5 minutes
- Cook Time: 20 minutes
- Total Time: 25 minutes
- Serving: 4

<u>Ingredients</u>

- 4 skinless, boneless chicken breast
- 2 tablespoons extra virgin olive oil, divided
- 1½ cups unsalted chicken stock (organic preferred)
- 2 skin-removed large potatoes
- ½ cup lactose-free milk
- 1 teaspoon black pepper, divided

- ¼ teaspoon salt, divided
- ¼ teaspoon turmeric
- 1 tablespoon minced parsley (optional)

<u>Preparation</u>

1. High-heat 2 tablespoons of extra virgin olive oil in a pan. Add your chicken breast with ½ tablespoon of salt, pepper, and one tablespoon of turmeric and let it cook until golden brown both sides.
2. Cook all potatoes in a medium pot with a little pinch of turmeric.
3. Mash your potatoes and add the rest of salt and pepper.
4. Heat lactose-free milk in the microwave and add to your mashed potato. Whisk well.
5. Pour your plate with mashed potato, and chicken on top.

<u>Cooking Tips:</u>

- You can make the Béchamel sauce (explained before in Fettuccine Alfredo recipe) and add it to your chicken and mashed potato.

<u>Fructose Intolerance-related Tips:</u>

- Do not use parsley if you cannot tolerate it.
- If you are in a flare, try not to use too much pepper.

Nutrition Facts

Servings: 4

Amount per serving

Calories	**448**
	% Daily Value*
Total Fat 15.8g	20%
Saturated Fat 3.1g	16%
Cholesterol 108mg	36%
Sodium 279mg	12%
Total Carbohydrate 33g	12%
Dietary Fiber 3.3g	12%
Total Sugars 3.1g	
Protein 42.8g	
Vitamin D 0mcg	0%
Calcium 49mg	4%
Iron 3mg	14%
Potassium 911mg	19%

CHICKEN STROGANOFF

Try Chicken Stroganoff with potatoes and incredible gravy, matched with patient's tolerance levels.

- Prep Time: 5 minutes
- Cook Time: 15 minutes
- Total Time: 20 minutes
- Serving: 4

<u>Ingredients</u>

- 4 skinless, boneless chicken breast
- 2 tablespoons gluten-free flour
- 2 cups (~500 ml) unsalted/salt-reduced beef broth (organic preferred)
- 1 tablespoon of salt and pepper
- 3 tablespoons extra virgin olive oil
- 1 tablespoon Dijon mustard
- ⅓ cup lactose-free milk
- 1 tablespoon fresh lemon juice
- ½ tablespoon ginseng powder or fresh ginseng
- ½ tablespoon turmeric
- ½ tsp garlic powder (optional)

- Parsley, minced (optional)

<u>Instructions</u>

1. Heat a tablespoon of high-quality extra virgin olive oil in a pan. Flat your chicken breasts and cook them with ½ tablespoon of salt, ½ tablespoon of pepper and ginseng powder until golden brown both sides.
2. In another pan, put one tablespoon of extra virgin olive oil on medium heat. Then, add your flour slowly and whisk until golden brown.
3. Heat your lactose-free milk in the microwave, add it slowly to your flour, and whisk for 3 minutes. Add lemon juice, garlic powder (optional), Dijon mustard, ½ tablespoon of pepper, and ½ tablespoon of salt to make a great sauce. Stir the sauce on low heat until it becomes thick.
4. Fry very thin-sliced potatoes with one tablespoon of extra virgin olive oil and ½ tablespoon of turmeric.
5. Add your fries and chicken to your sauce. Let it cook for two more minutes.
6. Garnish the top with minced parsley and enjoy!

<u>Cooking Tips:</u>

- You can use pork tenderloin or turkey breast instead of chicken breast.

<u>Fructose Intolerance-related Tips:</u>

- If you are in a flare-up, try not to use pepper.
- Do not use parsley if you cannot tolerate them.

Nutrition Facts	
Servings: 4	
Amount per serving	
Calories	**274**
	% Daily Value*
Total Fat 13.2g	17%
Saturated Fat 1.9g	10%
Cholesterol 67mg	22%
Sodium 433mg	19%
Total Carbohydrate 10.7g	4%
Dietary Fiber 2.6g	9%
Total Sugars 2.7g	
Protein 29.8g	
Vitamin D 15mcg	77%
Calcium 42mg	3%
Iron 3mg	17%
Potassium 331mg	7%

Chicken Kebab

Enjoy a classic barbecued chicken, well-marinated in saffron and yogurt!

- Prep Time: 15 minutes
- (Marinate Time: 2 hours)
- Cook Time: 25 minutes
- Total Time: 40 minutes
- Serving: 4

Ingredients

- 4 chicken breasts, cut into 1.5 inches (3.8) cubes
- ¾ cup lactose-free yogurt
- 1 large onion
- ¼ cup saffron (bloomed)
- 1 tablespoon salt
- 3 tablespoons extra virgin olive oil
- 1 tablespoon lemon juice

Instructions

1. Cut your onions and make onion rings.

2. To marinate your chicken, mix and stir it well with onion, lactose-free plain yogurt, bloomed saffron, olive oil, salt, and lemon juice together (To have a bloomed saffron, you need to grind your saffron perfectly and add 100ml of boiling water to it).

3. Cover the marinated bowl and put it in the fridge to rest for two hours.

4. After two hours, thread chickens into skewers and grilled both sides well until golden brown

<u>Cooking Tips:</u>

- You can use the oven instead of grilling chickens. Just preheat the oven to 400 °F, cover chickens with aluminum foils, and let it cook for about 25 minutes. Use broil for five minutes if you want a golden brown texture.

- You can use chicken with bones instead of chicken breasts, as well.

<u>Fructose Intolerance-related Tips:</u>

- If you cannot tolerate saffron (rarely happens), do not add saffron to chicken. Instead, put ⅓ tablespoon of turmeric.

Nutrition Facts

Servings: 4

Amount per serving

Calories   **322**

	% Daily Value*
Total Fat 21g	27%
Saturated Fat 2.5g	12%
Cholesterol 68mg	23%
Sodium 1812mg	79%
Total Carbohydrate 7.4g	3%
Dietary Fiber 0.9g	3%
Total Sugars 1.7g	
Protein 27.6g	
Vitamin D 0mcg	0%
Calcium 70mg	5%
Iron 0mg	2%
Potassium 174mg	4%

ROASTED CHICKEN WITH POMEGRANATE SAUCE

Have you tried a sour taste of chicken with pomegranate sauce? This dish is an excellent sample of a delicious sour chicken. You can make your dish sweet and sour by adding brown sugar to the recipe.

- Prep Time: 10 minutes
- (Marinate Time: 2 hours)
- Cook Time: 40 minutes
- Total Time: 50 minutes
- Serving: 4

<u>Ingredients</u>

- 4 Chicken legs and thighs, skinless
- ¼ cup bloomed saffron
- 2 tablespoons extra virgin olive oil
- 5 tablespoons lime juice
- ½ cup pomegranate sauce
- 1 tablespoon salt
- 1 tablespoon turmeric
- 2 cups of water
- ½ tablespoon black pepper

- ½ cup brown sugar (optional)

Instructions

1. In a large bowl, marinate your chicken with bloomed saffron, lime juice, brown sugar (optional) salt and pepper.
2. Mix and stir all ingredients well. Cover the bowl top and fridge it for 2 hours.
3. Roast your chicken with extra virgin olive oil and turmeric for 15 minutes until golden brown.
4. Boil two cups of water and add pomegranate sauce. Stir well until dissolved.
5. Put your chicken in the sauce and let it cook for 25 minutes. Let the sauce thicken, and then you are done!
6. Serve it with white basmati rice and enjoy!

Cooking Tips:

- Alternatively, you may want to use chicken breasts instead of chicken legs and thighs.
- If you do not find the pomegranate sauce or paste, you can add 200ml of pomegranate juice. It makes your meal hard to be thickened, but it gives you a similar taste.

Fructose Intolerance-related Tips:

- If you cannot tolerate saffron (rarely happens), do not add saffron to chicken. Instead, put ⅓ tablespoon of turmeric.
- Pomegranate has anti-inflammatory properties, which is excellent for people with fructose

intolerance, and it can be well-tolerate in many patients.

Nutrition Facts	
Servings: 4	
Amount per serving	
Calories	**303**
	% Daily Value*
Total Fat 17.2g	22%
Saturated Fat 3.6g	18%
Cholesterol 90mg	30%
Sodium 2094mg	91%
Total Carbohydrate 16.4g	6%
Dietary Fiber 0.6g	2%
Total Sugars 11.4g	
Protein 22.7g	
Vitamin D 0mcg	0%
Calcium 33mg	3%
Iron 2mg	13%
Potassium 79mg	2%

PUFFY CHICKEN

A tremendous yummy puffy chicken strips for adults and kids.

- Prep Time: 10 minutes
- Cook Time: 20 minutes
- Total Time: 30 minutes
- Serving: 4

<u>Ingredients</u>

- 4 strip cuts of chicken breast (~400 grams)
- 150 grams of gluten-free flour
- 5 tablespoons alcohol-free carbonated malt drink
- 2 tablespoons extra virgin olive oil
- 3 eggs (organic range-free preferred)
- 1 tablespoon Dijon mustard
- ½ tablespoon salt
- ½ tablespoon turmeric powder
- ½ teaspoon brown sugar (optional)

- 1 tablespoon active dried yeast (optional)

Instructions

1. In a large bowl, marinate your chicken with malt drink, yeast, olive oil, mustard, salt, and turmeric. Mix all well.
2. In another bowl, whisk all three eggs perfectly.
3. First, deep your marinated chickens into eggs and then cover it with flour.
4. Cook your chicken in a pan over medium heat with extra virgin olive oil.

Cooking Tips:

- You can use brown sugar to give a sweet taste to your dish.
- Instead of carbonated malt drink, you can use carbonated water. In this case, you need to use active dry yeast.

Fructose Intolerance-related Tips:

- If you can tolerate beer a little bit, you can use it instead of malt drink.
- This dish is well-matched with Tartar sauce. So, if you tolerate Tartar, enjoy this meal with it!

Nutrition Facts	
Servings: 4	
Amount per serving	
Calories	**458**
	% Daily Value*
Total Fat 16g	20%
Saturated Fat 3.5g	18%
Cholesterol 221mg	74%
Sodium 1051mg	46%
Total Carbohydrate 31.8g	12%
Dietary Fiber 1.3g	5%
Total Sugars 2g	
Protein 44.3g	
Vitamin D 12mcg	58%
Calcium 46mg	4%
Iron 4mg	22%
Potassium 410mg	9%

CHICKEN SCALOPPINI

Enjoy a delicious Italian dish with ingredients great for people with fructose intolerance!

- Prep Time: 10 minutes
- Cook Time: 15 minutes
- Total Time: 25 minutes
- Serving: 4

<u>Ingredients</u>

- 4 skinless and boneless chicken breast
- 2 teaspoons fresh lemon juice
- 1 tablespoon extra virgin olive oil
- 6 tablespoons gluten-free bread crumbs or any gluten-free dried bread
- ½ cup unsalted, no-fat chicken broth
- 1 tablespoon lime juice
- 1 tablespoon well-cooked capers
- ¼ teaspoon salt
- ¼ teaspoon black pepper
- ¼ cup grape vinegar (optional)

<u>Instructions</u>

1. First, use a meat mallet to pound your chicken breasts.
2. Add lemon juice, salt, and pepper to your chicken
3. Heat a pan with extra virgin olive oil over medium heat. Add your chicken to the pan and cook each side for about 5 minutes until golden brown.
4. In the end, add chicken broth, grape vinegar (optional), and your breadcrumbs and stir well for five more minutes until it gets thick.
5. Garnish with capers. Enjoy!

<u>Cooking Tips:</u>

- You can use sour grape juice or grape vinegar if you want to give a bitter taste to your meal only if you tolerate them.

<u>Fructose Intolerance-related Tips:</u>

- If you can tolerate sour grape juice or grape vinegar, you can add it to your broth.
- Make sure you cooked capers well.

Nutrition Facts

Servings: 4

Amount per serving

Calories	320
	% Daily Value*
Total Fat 11g	14%
Saturated Fat 2.6g	13%
Cholesterol 35mg	12%
Sodium 863mg	38%
Total Carbohydrate 33.2g	12%
Dietary Fiber 1.5g	6%
Total Sugars 0.7g	
Protein 20.6g	
Vitamin D 0mcg	0%
Calcium 19mg	1%
Iron 2mg	9%
Potassium 28mg	1%

CHICKEN-PINEAPPLE PIZZA

Do you think lactose-intolerant patients cannot eat pizza anymore? You might be wrong! Try this recipe to have a great pizza taste!

- Prep Time: 10 minutes
- Cook Time: 15 minutes
- Total Time: 25 minutes
- Serving: 4

<u>Ingredients</u>

- 4 gluten-free pizza crusts
- 1 cup sliced no-fat cooked chicken breast
- 1 cup pineapple chunks
- 1 cup shredded lactose-free mozzarella cheese
- 4 tablespoons organic mayonnaise
- 1 teaspoon oregano powder

<u>Instructions</u>

1. Place your gluten-free pizza crusts on a non-stick pizza pan or bake sheet.
2. Spread your organic low-fat low-sodium mayo on your crust.
3. Add your cooked chicken breasts and pineapple to your pizza
4. Sprinkle with lactose-free cheese
5. Let it bake at 480 °F for 10 minutes. Then, broil on the same heat for five more minutes until cheese melted.

<u>Cooking Tips:</u>

- You can use any other white sauces such as béchamel sauce instead of mayo.

<u>Fructose Intolerance-related Tips:</u>

- If you are lactose intolerant, use lactose-free or dairy-free cheese for pizza
- Use mayonnaise only if you can tolerate it. If you cannot tolerate, you can make a béchamel sauce instead (explained before in Fettuccine Alfredo recipe).

Nutrition Facts

Servings: 4

Amount per serving

Calories	**342**

	% Daily Value*
Total Fat 12.4g	16%
Saturated Fat 2.7g	14%
Cholesterol 47mg	16%
Sodium 499mg	22%
Total Carbohydrate 39.1g	14%
Dietary Fiber 2.1g	7%
Total Sugars 7g	
Protein 18.5g	
Vitamin D 0mcg	0%
Calcium 82mg	6%
Iron 1mg	7%
Potassium 165mg	4%

TURKEY ZUCCHINI NOODLES

If you look for a healthy meal for your lunch or dinner, you can try Turkey Zucchini Noodles. If you have some leftover turkeys from Thanksgiving or any other events, it would be an excellent option for you to cook this delicious main course.

- Prep Time: 15 minutes
- Cook Time: 15 minutes
- Total Time: 30 minutes
- Serving: 4

<u>Ingredients</u>

- 3 medium-size spiralized zucchinis or zucchini strips
- 1 lb (~455 g) skinless fat-free cooked turkey breasts

- 1 tablespoon extra virgin olive oil, divided
- 2 cups of water
- ½ teaspoon turmeric
- ½ teaspoon salt
- 1 tablespoon tomato paste (optional)

Instructions

1. Cook zucchini noodles in boiling water for 5 minutes.
2. Bring them out of the water and let them dry.
3. Heat your cooked turkey in a pan with extra virgin olive oil. Add turmeric, tomato paste (optional), salt, and little water (~100ml) for 5 minutes until golden brown both sides.
4. Add your zucchini to your turkey and stir well. Enjoy!

Cooking Tips:

- You can use a can of organic crushed tomatoes instead of tomato paste if you can tolerate them.

Fructose Intolerance-related Tips:

- Consume organic tomato paste in moderation or remove it from the recipe.

Nutrition Facts

Servings: 4

Amount per serving

Calories	172
	% Daily Value*
Total Fat 5.7g	7%
Saturated Fat 0.9g	5%
Cholesterol 49mg	16%
Sodium 1460mg	63%
Total Carbohydrate 9.9g	4%
Dietary Fiber 2.3g	8%
Total Sugars 6.5g	
Protein 21.2g	
Vitamin D 0mcg	0%
Calcium 35mg	3%
Iron 2mg	13%
Potassium 736mg	16%

ZUCCHINI EGG DISH

Are you looking for a vegetarian dish that is well-matched with fructose intolerance diet? Try a fabulous Zucchini Egg dish.

- Prep Time: 10 minutes
- Cook Time: 15 minutes
- Total Time: 25 minutes
- Serving: 4

<u>Ingredients</u>

- 3 medium-size, diced zucchinis
- 2 organic range-free eggs
- 1 tablespoon garlic powder (optional)
- 1 tablespoon extra virgin olive oil
- ½ teaspoon turmeric powder
- ½ teaspoon salt
- ½ teaspoon black pepper

<u>Instructions</u>

1. Peels off zucchinis and cook them in a pan over medium heat.
2. When zucchinis become soft, flattened them or blend them in a blender.
3. Add garlic powder, turmeric, salt, and pepper to your pan.
4. Whisk eggs in a small bowl and add them to your zucchinis.
5. When the eggs get coagulate, mix them with your zucchinis. Enjoy!

<u>Cooking Tips:</u>

- You can also add one tablespoon of tomato paste if you can tolerate it.

<u>Fructose Intolerance-related Tips:</u>

- Do not use black pepper in your meal if you are in a severe flare-up.

Nutrition Facts

Servings: 4

Amount per serving	
Calories	**94**
	% Daily Value*
Total Fat 6g	8%
Saturated Fat 1.2g	6%
Cholesterol 82mg	27%
Sodium 337mg	15%
Total Carbohydrate 7g	3%
Dietary Fiber 2g	7%
Total Sugars 3.2g	
Protein 5g	
Vitamin D 8mcg	39%
Calcium 37mg	3%
Iron 1mg	7%
Potassium 448mg	10%

POTATO CUTLET

Potato Cutlet is an easy to cook vegetarian recipe for people with fructose intolerance with a yummy crispy texture.

- Prep Time: 10 minutes
- Cook Time: 20 minutes
- Total Time: 30 minutes
- Serving: 4

<u>Ingredients</u>

- 2 lbs yellow skin-removed potatoes
- 5 large organic range-free eggs
- 3 tablespoons extra virgin olive oil
- ½ teaspoon turmeric powder

- Salt and black pepper to taste

<u>Instructions</u>

1. Remove potato skins and scrub potatoes with a scrubber.
2. In a large bowl, mix potatoes and all other ingredients perfectly.
3. Make potato cutlets by rounding-and-flattening them in your hand.
4. Heat your high-quality extra virgin olive oil in a skillet over medium heat. Add your cutlets to the pan and flatten them.
5. Let it cook each side until golden brown.

<u>Cooking Tips:</u>

- You can add one teaspoon freshly grated ginseng to your ingredients, as well.

<u>Fructose Intolerance-related Tips:</u>

- Do not use black pepper in your meal if you are in a severe flare-up.

Nutrition Facts

Servings: 4

Amount per serving

Calories	273
	% Daily Value*
Total Fat 10.6g	14%
Saturated Fat 1.5g	8%
Cholesterol 0mg	0%
Sodium 112mg	5%
Total Carbohydrate 40.5g	15%
Dietary Fiber 4.1g	15%
Total Sugars 2.3g	
Protein 8.5g	
Vitamin D 0mcg	0%
Calcium 164mg	13%
Iron 2mg	13%
Potassium 75mg	2%

GINSENG STICKY PORK

Are you looking for a satisfying, easy to cook a meal with pork? Ginseng Sticky Pork is a great candidate for you and your family members with fructose intolerance.

- Prep Time: 15 minutes
- Cook Time: 10 minutes
- Total Time: 25 minutes
- Serving: 6

<u>Ingredients</u>

- 1½ lb boneless, fat-removed pork tenderloin, cut into strips with ½ inch (~1.3cm) thickness
- 1 tablespoon extra virgin olive oil
- ½ cup brown sugar
- 2 inches (~5cm) fresh ginseng knob
- 1 tablespoon lemon juice
- 1 teaspoon salt
- ½ teaspoon black pepper
- 1 tablespoon garlic powder (optional)
- 1 tablespoon grape vinegar (optional)

<u>Instructions</u>

1. Heat extra virgin olive oil in a skillet over medium-high heat until shimmering.
2. Add your pork, salt, and pepper to the skillet. Brown one side first and then brown the other side of pork. Take out your pork.
3. Add ginseng, lemon juice, grape vinegar (optional), garlic powder (optional), and brown sugar to the pan. Stir and bring to boil.

4. When the sauce gets thick and sticky, bring back your pork. Enjoy!

<u>Cooking Tips:</u>

- This dish can be served perfectly with white steamed rice.

<u>Fructose Intolerance-related Tips:</u>

- Do not use black pepper in your meal if you are in a severe flare-up.

Nutrition Facts	
Servings: 6	
Amount per serving	
Calories	**275**
	% Daily Value*
Total Fat 6.4g	8%
Saturated Fat 1.7g	9%
Cholesterol 83mg	28%
Sodium 454mg	20%
Total Carbohydrate 24.9g	9%
Dietary Fiber 0.4g	1%
Total Sugars 23.5g	
Protein 30g	
Vitamin D 0mcg	0%
Calcium 12mg	1%
Iron 2mg	9%
Potassium 521mg	11%

GERMAN PORK SCHNITZEL

If you are looking for tender pork with a crispy crust, try German Pork Schnitzel. It is very easy to make it, and it is well-matched with baby carrots and potato garnishes.

- Prep Time: 20 minutes
- Cook Time: 15 minutes
- Total Time: 35 minutes
- Serving: 4

<u>Ingredients</u>

- 2 lbs boneless fatless pork tenderloins flattened into ½ inch (1.3cm) thick
- 3 large organic free-range eggs
- 2 cups gluten-free bread crumbs
- ⅓ cup gluten-free flour
- 2 tablespoons extra virgin olive oil
- Lemon wedges for taste
- ½ teaspoon salt
- ½ teaspoon black pepper

<u>Instructions</u>

1. Pound your pork pieces with a mallet until it gets ½ inch thick.
2. In a medium bowl, mix flour, and pepper.
3. In another bowl, whisk three eggs.
4. In another bowl or plate, spread your breadcrumbs.
5. First, put both sides of pork cutlets in flour. Then, dip them in egg and then drip them into breadcrumbs using a fork.
6. Now, heat a large pan with extra virgin olive oil over medium heat. When the oil gets very hot, cook your cutlets for 5 minutes, each side until each side gets golden brown.
7. Enjoy the meal with lemon wedges!

<u>Cooking Tips:</u>

- This dish can be served perfectly with mashed potatoes. If you are lactose-intolerant, use lactose-free milk to make mashed potatoes.

<u>Fructose Intolerance-related Tips:</u>

- Do not use black pepper in your meal if you are in a severe flare-up.

Nutrition Facts

Servings: 4	
Amount per serving	
Calories	**600**
	% Daily Value*
Total Fat 19.3g	25%
Saturated Fat 4.7g	23%
Cholesterol 243mg	81%
Sodium 979mg	43%
Total Carbohydrate 49.6g	18%
Dietary Fiber 2.9g	10%
Total Sugars 5.7g	
Protein 54.5g	
Vitamin D 12mcg	58%
Calcium 120mg	9%
Iron 6mg	33%
Potassium 169mg	4%

PINEAPPLE PORK

A delicious pork-based recipe that has been modified for people with fructose intolerance.

- Prep Time: 5 minutes
- Cook Time: 25 minutes
- Total Time: 30 minutes
- Serving: 4

Ingredients

- 2 lbs skinless, boneless pork tenderloin
- 1 cup small pineapple, cut into small cubes
- 1 tablespoon peeled and grated ginseng (~1 inch or ~2.5 cm)
- 1 tablespoons soy sauce (optional)
- 2 tablespoons balsamic vinegar
- 2 tablespoons extra virgin olive oil
- Salt and black pepper to taste
- 1 teaspoon garlic powder (optional)

<u>Instructions</u>

1. Mix ginseng, garlic powder (optional), balsamic vinegar, and soy sauce in a small bowl.
2. Add salt and pepper to your pork.
3. Use a large skillet and cook both sides of your pork in it over medium heat with high-quality extra virgin olive oil until golden brown.
4. Check by a knife to see if the inside pork cooked or not. Remove the pork pieces from the skillet. Add your sauce to the pan and let it cooked for three more minutes.
5. Cook your pineapple in the same skillet for three minutes. If the sauce gets dry, add a little bit of water.
6. Bring back pork pieces to the skillet and let it cook for one more minute.

<u>Cooking Tips:</u>

- This dish can be served with steamed white rice.
- You can use peeled and poached peach cubes instead of pineapple.

<u>Fructose Intolerance-related Tips:</u>

- Do not use black pepper or garlic powder if you are experiencing a severe flare-up.
- Vinegar may reduce inflammation in the colon. However, its sourness can annoy your gut. Try to use less vinegar if you are in a flare-up.
- Use soy sauce only if you can tolerate it. Remove it from the recipe if it irritates you.

Nutrition Facts
Servings: 4

Amount per serving

Calories   **375**

	% Daily Value*
Total Fat 15.2g	19%
Saturated Fat 4g	20%
Cholesterol 132mg	44%
Sodium 533mg	23%
Total Carbohydrate 7.4g	3%
Dietary Fiber 0.7g	2%
Total Sugars 5.5g	
Protein 51.3g	
Vitamin D 0mcg	0%
Calcium 7mg	1%
Iron 2mg	10%
Potassium 68mg	1%

BALSAMIC-PEACH PORK

Balsamic-Peach Pork is a great and easy-to-cook meal with few ingredients. A fantastic combination of peach and brown sugar gives the dish a lovely sweet taste.

- Prep Time: 10 minutes
- Cook Time: 20 minutes
- Total Time: 30 minutes
- Serving: 4

Ingredients

- 2 boneless pork tenderloins
- 1 sliced peeled peach
- 6 oz lactose-free Swiss cheese
- ½ cup balsamic vinegar
- 1 tablespoon brown sugar
- 2 tablespoons extra virgin olive oil
- 1 tablespoon fresh chopped oregano or thyme leaves
- Salt and black pepper to taste
- ½ cup fresh basil (optional)

Instructions

1. Mix cheese, balsamic vinegar, brown sugar, oregano, or thyme leaves in a bowl.
2. Add salt and pepper to your pork.
3. Use a large skillet and cook both sides of your pork in it over medium heat with high-quality extra virgin olive oil until golden brown.
4. Check by knife if inside pork cooked well. Remove the pork pieces from the skillet. Add your sauce to the pan and let it cooked for three more minutes.
5. Cook your peeled-off peach in the same skillet for five minutes. If your sauce gets dry, add water a little bit.
6. Bring back pork pieces to the skillet and let it cook for two more minutes.
7. Garnish with fresh basil if you want. Enjoy!

<u>Cooking Tips:</u>

- This dish can be served well with steamed white rice.
- You can have lactose-free Havarti cheese instead of Swiss cheese.

<u>Fructose Intolerance-related Tips:</u>

- Peach may irritate your gut. That is why this recipe only uses one peach. Limit taking peach or poach it if you cannot tolerate it.
- Do not use black pepper or lots of green basils if you are experiencing a severe flare-up.
- Vinegar can reduce inflammation in the colon. However, its sourness can annoy your gut. Try to use less vinegar if you are in a flare-up.

Nutrition Facts

Servings: 4

Amount per serving

Calories | **266**

	% Daily Value*
Total Fat 15.6g	20%
Saturated Fat 1.5g	8%
Cholesterol 31mg	10%
Sodium 476mg	21%
Total Carbohydrate 14.6g	5%
Dietary Fiber 1.7g	6%
Total Sugars 11.5g	
Protein 18.7g	
Vitamin D 1mcg	6%
Calcium 585mg	45%
Iron 2mg	11%
Potassium 365mg	8%

TURMERIC PORK

If you are looking for a healthy dish, you are reading the right recipe. A short cooking-time Turmeric Pork is an excellent choice for people with fructose intolerance who wants to have a rich pork-based main course.

- Prep Time: 15 minutes
- Cook Time: 15 minutes
- Total Time: 30 minutes
- Serving: 4

<u>Ingredients</u>

- 1¼ pounds chopped boneless, fat-removed pork tenderloin
- ½ cup plain lactose-free yogurt
- ¼ cup brown sugar
- 2 tablespoons extra virgin olive oil
- 3 small carrots
- 1½ teaspoons turmeric powder
- 3 tablespoons fresh lemon juice
- Salt and black pepper to taste
- 1 teaspoon garlic powder (optional)

<u>Instructions</u>

1. Mix plain yogurt, brown sugar, garlic powder (optional), turmeric, and lemon juice in a bowl.
2. Pour salt and pepper on your pork.
3. Use a large skillet and cook both sides of your pork in it over medium heat with high-quality extra virgin olive oil until golden brown.
4. Check by knife if inside pork cooked well. Remove the pork pieces from the skillet. Add your sauce to the pan and let it cooked for three more minutes.
5. Cook your carrots in a small skillet for 10 minutes as sides.
6. Bring back pork pieces to the skillet and let it cook for two more minutes. Enjoy!

<u>Cooking Tips:</u>

- This dish can be served well with steamed white rice or noodles.

Nutrition Facts

Servings: 4

Amount per serving

Calories	624

	% Daily Value*
Total Fat 18.7g	24%
Saturated Fat 5.2g	26%
Cholesterol 229mg	76%
Sodium 235mg	10%
Total Carbohydrate 26.4g	10%
Dietary Fiber 1.9g	7%
Total Sugars 22.2g	
Protein 84.1g	
Vitamin D 0mcg	0%
Calcium 98mg	8%
Iron 5mg	26%
Potassium 1633mg	35%

GRILLED LEAN BEEF KEBAB

Extra-lean beef with no fats is recommended for people with fructose intolerance who want to consume red meats.

Another fabulous alternative to red meat is Ostrich meat. It tastes very similar to lean beef, but it has less fat, cholesterol. It is high in calcium, iron, and protein. It is highly recommended for people with fructose intolerance to include Ostrich beef in their diet once a week.

- Prep Time: 10 minutes
- Marinate Time: 60 minutes
- Cook Time: 20 minutes
- Total Time: 90 minutes
- Serving: 4

Ingredients

- 2 lbs extra lean beef or lamb meat
- ½ cup plain lactose-free yogurt
- 1 small kiwi
- 1 onion (thinly sliced)
- 1 tablespoon extra virgin olive oil
- 4 tablespoons fresh lemon juice
- Salt and black pepper to taste

Instructions

1. Cut extra lean beef/lamb into small 1-inch (~2.54cm) cubes.
2. Ina large bowl, marinate your beef/lamb with plain yogurt, onion, kiwi, lemon juice, olive oil, salt, and pepper.
3. Cover the top bowl, fridge it and Let it marinate for 1 hour.
4. Skewer your kebab cubes or just grill both sides like a steak. Ten minutes grill would suffice for medium kebabs, and 20 minutes grill would suffice for well-done kebabs.

<u>Cooking Tips:</u>

- You do not necessarily need to cut your beef/lamb into cubes. You can flatten them by mallet and make a fantastic steak.
- Make sure you remove all onion slices that are stuck to your kebab skewers.
- Kiwi melts your kebab and makes it very juicy.
- This dish can be served well with steamed white rice.

<u>Fructose Intolerance-related Tips:</u>

- Do not use black pepper or onion if you are experiencing a severe flare-up.

Nutrition Facts	
Servings: 4	
Amount per serving	
Calories	**499**
	% Daily Value*
Total Fat 18.3g	23%
Saturated Fat 6.3g	31%
Cholesterol 205mg	68%
Sodium 176mg	8%
Total Carbohydrate 7.9g	3%
Dietary Fiber 1.2g	4%
Total Sugars 5.4g	
Protein 71.2g	
Vitamin D 0mcg	0%
Calcium 73mg	6%
Iron 43mg	238%
Potassium 1104mg	23%

HUNGARIAN GOULASH

Goulash is a great traditional stew full of healthy ingredients. People with fructose intolerance need to add more bone, beef, chicken, or vegetable broth meals in their diet. Hungarian Goulash is a great option that can be added to your weekly meal plan.

- Prep Time: 30 minutes
- Cook Time: 90 minutes

- Total Time: 120 minutes
- Serving: 6

Ingredients

- 1½ lbs extra lean beef trimmed into 1 inch (~2.54 cm) cubes
- 2 cups bone/beef broth or tap water
- 2 tablespoons extra virgin olive oil
- 2 tablespoons lemon juice
- ½ tablespoon turmeric
- 1 teaspoon salt
- ¼ teaspoon pepper
- 1 cup carrots
- 2 cups potatoes, cut into 1 inch (~2.54cm) cubes
- 1 tablespoon tomato paste (optional)

Instructions

1. One a large pan or a pot, heat olive oil, turmeric, tomato paste (optional), and pepper over medium heat.
2. Add your extra lean beef and stir for 5 minutes.
3. Add water or bone/beef broth slowly to your pot. Then, cover and let it cook for 50 minutes over low heat until tender.
4. Add potatoes and let it cook for 20 more minutes. Add salt and lemon juice. Then, add the carrots and cook the stew for 15 more minutes. Enjoy!

Cooking Tips:

- This dish can be served well with steamed white rice.
- Anytime the stew gets very thick, add more water into it.

<u>Fructose Intolerance-related Tips:</u>

- Do not use black pepper or tomato paste if you are experiencing a severe flare-up.

Nutrition Facts
Servings: 6

Amount per serving	
Calories	**309**
	% Daily Value*
Total Fat 12.4g	16%
Saturated Fat 3.5g	18%
Cholesterol 101mg	34%
Sodium 734mg	32%
Total Carbohydrate 10.5g	4%
Dietary Fiber 1.8g	6%
Total Sugars 1.8g	
Protein 37.1g	
Vitamin D 0mcg	0%
Calcium 17mg	1%
Iron 22mg	123%
Potassium 810mg	17%

TOMATO FREE SPAGHETTI BOLOGNESE

Many of people with fructose intolerance cannot well-tolerated tomatoes and tomato pastes, which can negatively affect their regular cooking habits using tomatoes inside meals. Let us try a great Spaghetti Bolognese tomato-free! Yes, you read correctly! Enjoy a tomato-free Italian dish now!

- Prep Time: 15 minutes
- Cook Time: 25 minutes
- Total Time: 40 minutes
- Serving: 4

<u>Ingredients</u>

- 1 lb (~500 s) extra lean ground beef
- 0.65 lb (~300 g) gluten-free spaghetti
- 1 cup organic unsalted chicken stock
- 1 tablespoon extra virgin olive oil
- 1 tablespoon soy sauce (optional)

- 2 tablespoons brown sugar
- 1 teaspoon dried oregano or oregano powder
- ½ teaspoon dried thyme
- 1 teaspoon dried basil
- ½ tablespoon turmeric
- 1 teaspoon salt
- ¼ teaspoon pepper
- 1 tablespoon lactose-free cheese (optional)

Instructions

1. Golden both sides of your extra lean ground beef in a large pan with extra virgin olive oil over high heat.
2. Add soy sauce, brown sugar, salt, pepper, turmeric, and chicken stock to your ground beef. Let it thicken and have it cooked for one more minute.
3. At the same time, prepare your spaghetti according to its package recipe with a pinch of salt and a little bit of olive oil.
4. Take your spaghetti out of boiling water and put it in your sauce.
5. Season it with dried basil and cheese.

Cooking Tips:

- If your sauce thickened more than desired, add some tap water or spaghetti boiling water.

Fructose Intolerance-related Tips:

- Do not use black pepper, Parmesan, or fresh herbs if you are experiencing a severe flare-up.

Nutrition Facts	
Servings: 4	
Amount per serving	
Calories	**475**
	% Daily Value*
Total Fat 12.9g	17%
Saturated Fat 4.2g	21%
Cholesterol 141mg	47%
Sodium 1092mg	47%
Total Carbohydrate 49.1g	18%
Dietary Fiber 0.5g	2%
Total Sugars 6.3g	
Protein 38.8g	
Vitamin D 0mcg	0%
Calcium 42mg	3%
Iron 7mg	37%
Potassium 593mg	13%

LAMB/BEEF LIVER STEW

A great stew with excellent sources of Iron, Vitamin A, D, and B12 for people with fructose intolerance.

- Prep Time: 10 minutes
- Cook Time: 20 minutes
- Total Time: 30 minutes
- Serving: 4

<u>Ingredients</u>

- 1 lb (~500 g) lamb/beef liver, cut in 1 inch (~2.54cm) cubes
- 1 cup of organic unsalted bone/beef broth
- 2 tablespoons extra virgin olive oil
- 2 teaspoons turmeric
- 1 teaspoon salt
- ½ teaspoon pepper
- 1 potato, cut into 1 inch (~2.54cm) cubes (optional)
- 2 tablespoons tomato paste (optional)

<u>Instructions</u>

1. Fully cook your lamb/beef liver in a large pan with extra virgin olive oil, turmeric, salt and pepper, potatoes (optional), and tomato paste (optional) over medium heat for 15 minutes.
2. Add your bone/beef broth to your livers. Cook for 5 minutes until thickened.

Cooking Tips:

- You can add 1 tablespoon of gluten-free flour if your stew is not getting thick.
- If your stew thickened more than desired, add some hot water to it.
- If you are in high cholesterol, you can substitute the liver with the extra lean ostrich.

Fructose Intolerance-related Tips:

- Do not use black pepper and tomato paste if you are experiencing a flare-up.

Nutrition Facts

Servings: 4

Amount per serving

Calories	273
	% Daily Value*
Total Fat 12.8g	16%
Saturated Fat 2.8g	14%
Cholesterol 432mg	144%
Sodium 860mg	37%
Total Carbohydrate 7g	3%
Dietary Fiber 0.3g	1%
Total Sugars 0.2g	
Protein 31.4g	
Vitamin D 0mcg	0%
Calcium 13mg	1%
Iron 8mg	43%
Potassium 481mg	10%

GRILLED SALMON

Try a yummy grilled salmon dish.

- Prep Time: 5 minutes
- Cook Time: 25 minutes
- Total Time: 30 minutes
- Serving: 4

Ingredients:

- 2 lbs (~1 kg) salmon fillets
- ¼ cup brown sugar
- 1 tablespoon extra virgin olive oil
- 1 teaspoon turmeric powder
- 1 tablespoon fresh thyme leaves
- Salt and black pepper, to taste
- 1 teaspoon garlic powder (optional)

Directions:

1. Choose a medium bowl and whisk brown sugar, turmeric, thyme leaves, garlic (optional), extra virgin olive oil, salt, and pepper together.
2. Preheat your oven to 375 °F.
3. Pour your sauce over the salmon.
4. Put your salmon in the oven and let it cook for 20 minutes (until inside cooks well).
5. Enjoy!

Cooking Tips:

- If your salmon is thicker, you have to increase the cooking time until inside cooks well.
- You can cover your salmon with foil for having a juicy texture.

Fructose Intolerance-related Tips:

- Do not use black pepper in your meal if you are experiencing a flare-up.

Nutrition Facts	
Servings: 4	
Amount per serving	
Calories	**398**
	% Daily Value*
Total Fat 17.6g	23%
Saturated Fat 2.5g	13%
Cholesterol 100mg	33%
Sodium 101mg	4%
Total Carbohydrate 18.3g	7%
Dietary Fiber 0.4g	2%
Total Sugars 17.4g	
Protein 44.2g	
Vitamin D 0mcg	0%
Calcium 95mg	7%
Iron 3mg	15%
Potassium 902mg	19%

OVEN-BASED SALMON AND POTATO

A great mix of salmon and oven-baked potatoes give you a joyful lunch or dinner meal!

- Prep Time: 5 minutes
- Cook Time: 25 minutes
- Total Time: 30 minutes
- Serving: 4

Ingredients

- 4 salmon filets, about 6 ounces each
- 2 medium potatoes, sliced into very thin chips
- 3 tablespoons extra-virgin olive oil, divided
- 2 oranges
- 2 lemons
- Salt and pepper to taste

Instructions

1. Choose a small bowl and whisk orange juice, lemon juice, 1 tablespoon of extra virgin olive oil, salt, and pepper all together to have a juicy sauce.
2. Marinate your salmon with the sauce.
3. Slice potatoes very thin. Drizzle potatoes with two tablespoons of extra virgin olive oil and a pinch of salt.
4. Preheat your oven to 375 °F.
5. Choose a long foil sheet, put potatoes first, and fill the top with your salmon. Close your foil and let the salmon cook for about 25 minutes until inside cooks well.
6. Enjoy!

Cooking Tips:

- If your salmon is very thick, you have to increase the cooking time until inside cooks well.
- Check both salmon and your potato to be cooked. If required, return your salmon and potato to the over for five more minutes until perfection.

Fructose Intolerance-related Tips:

- Do not use black pepper in your meal if you are experiencing a flare-up.
- If you cannot tolerate orange juice, remove it from the recipe.

Nutrition Facts

Servings: 4

Amount per serving	
Calories	**443**
	% Daily Value*
Total Fat 21.8g	28%
Saturated Fat 3.1g	16%
Cholesterol 78mg	26%
Sodium 84mg	4%
Total Carbohydrate 28.4g	10%
Dietary Fiber 4.9g	18%
Total Sugars 10g	
Protein 37.4g	
Vitamin D 0mcg	0%
Calcium 117mg	9%
Iron 2mg	11%
Potassium 1248mg	27%

LEMON STEAMED HALIBUT WITH WHITE RICE

A great dish with healthy ingredients for people with fructose intolerance. You can substitute halibut with any other fishes you would like to have.

- Prep Time: 10 minutes
- Cook Time: 30 minutes
- Total Time: 40 minutes
- Serving: 6

<u>Ingredients</u>

- 6 skinless and boneless halibut fillets, about 6 ounces each
- 2 cups steamed white rice
- 1 tablespoon extra virgin olive oil
- 1 lemon, sliced very thin
- 4 tablespoons lemon juice
- 1 teaspoon ginseng powder
- Salt and pepper to taste
- Lemon wedges to garnish
- 1 teaspoon garlic powder (optional)

<u>Instructions</u>

1. Choose a small bowl and whisk lemon juice, ginseng powder, garlic powder (optional), extra virgin olive oil, salt, and pepper all together to have a juicy sauce.
2. Marinate your halibut with the sauce.
3. Preheat your oven to 375 °F.
4. Choose a long foil sheet, put halibut in your foil sheet, and close it. Let it cook for about 25 minutes until inside cooks well.
5. Open the foil sheet, put thin lemon slices on top of your halibut for 5 minutes, and close the foil sheet again.
6. Steam your white rice. Open your foil sheet and put halibut on top of the rice.
7. Garnish with lemon wedges. Enjoy!

<u>Cooking Tips:</u>

- If your halibut is very thick, you have to increase the cooking time until inside cooks well.

<u>Fructose Intolerance-related Tips:</u>

- Do not use black pepper in your meal if you are experiencing a flare-up.
- Do not use garlic powder if you cannot tolerate it.

Nutrition Facts	
Servings: 6	
Amount per serving	
Calories	**568**
	% Daily Value*
Total Fat 9.5g	12%
Saturated Fat 1.4g	7%
Cholesterol 93mg	31%
Sodium 161mg	7%
Total Carbohydrate 50.2g	18%
Dietary Fiber 1.3g	4%
Total Sugars 0.3g	
Protein 65g	
Vitamin D 0mcg	0%
Calcium 33mg	3%
Iron 16mg	87%
Potassium 1396mg	30%

THUNFISCH PIZZA

Thunfisch Pizza is an excellent German-based pizza with Tuna. The classic recipe has been modified to be tolerated by most people with fructose intolerance.

- Prep Time: 5 minutes
- Cook Time: 15 minutes
- Total Time: 20 minutes
- Serving: 4

Ingredients

- 2 medium-size gluten-free pizza crusts
- 1 cup shredded lactose-free cheese pizza
- Two 6.5 oz tuna can on oil or water
- 2 tablespoons organic mayonnaise
- 2 teaspoons dried ground oregano
- Salt to taste

Instructions

1. Place your gluten-free pizza crusts on a non-stick pizza pan or bake sheet.
2. Spread your organic mayo on your crust.

3. Gently put tuna on your pizza crust.
4. Sprinkle with lactose-free cheese
5. Let it bake at 400 °F for 10 minutes. Then, broil on the same heat for five more minutes until cheese melted.

<u>Cooking Tips:</u>

- You can use any other white sauces such as a béchamel sauce (explained before in Fettuccine Alfredo recipe) instead of mayonnaise.

<u>Fructose Intolerance-related Tips:</u>

- Use mayonnaise only if you can tolerate it. If you cannot tolerate, you can make a béchamel sauce (explain before in Fettuccine Alfredo recipe) instead.

Nutrition Facts	
Servings: 4	
Amount per serving	
Calories	**297**
	% Daily Value*
Total Fat 13g	17%
Saturated Fat 2.9g	14%
Cholesterol 33mg	11%
Sodium 333mg	14%
Total Carbohydrate 17g	6%
Dietary Fiber 0.8g	3%
Total Sugars 1.5g	
Protein 26.8g	
Vitamin D 0mcg	0%
Calcium 21mg	2%
Iron 1mg	5%
Potassium 310mg	7%

AVOCADO TUNA PITA

A very fast sandwich you can prepare at home for your lunch or dinner. You can even have a smaller portion of avocado tuna as a breakfast or as a snack at work.

- Prep Time: 10 minutes
- Cook Time: 0 minutes

- Total Time: 10 minutes
- Serving: 4

<u>Ingredients</u>

- 2 avocados
- 2 tablespoons organic mayonnaise
- 1 teaspoon cumin powder
- 1 can of tuna in olive oil or water
- 4 Pita bread or any gluten-free bread
- 1 teaspoon Dijon mustard (optional)
- Salt to taste
- Pepper to taste (optional)

<u>Instructions</u>

1. Choose a small bowl. Mix tuna with smashed avocado with mayo, cumin powder, mustard (optional), salt, and pepper (optional).
2. Open each of your pita bread from the corner and spoon the mix inside.
3. Roll the pita. Enjoy!

<u>Cooking Tips:</u>

- You can make this sandwich without mayonnaise sauce, as well.

<u>Fructose Intolerance-related Tips:</u>

- Do not use black pepper, cumin powder, or mustard if you are experiencing a flare-up.
- Always eat avocado in moderation.

Nutrition Facts	
Servings: 4	
Amount per serving	
Calories	**491**
	% Daily Value*
Total Fat 26.5g	34%
Saturated Fat 5.3g	27%
Cholesterol 16mg	5%
Sodium 442mg	19%
Total Carbohydrate 46g	17%
Dietary Fiber 8.5g	30%
Total Sugars 3.2g	
Protein 19.4g	
Vitamin D 0mcg	0%
Calcium 71mg	5%
Iron 3mg	16%
Potassium 733mg	16%

TROUT WITH ORANGE

Great classic seafood that typically serves with steamed white rice. It is recommended to make this dish with bitter or blood oranges.

- Prep Time: 20 minutes
- Cook Time: 30 minutes
- Total Time: 50 minutes
- Serving: 6

Ingredients

- Large fresh trout, 1.5 lbs each
- 3 oranges
- 1 tablespoon lemon juice
- 1 tablespoon extra virgin olive oil
- ½ teaspoon turmeric powder
- Salt & pepper to taste
- 1 teaspoon garlic powder (optional)

Instructions

1. Choose a medium bowl and whisk lemon juice, orange juice, turmeric powder, garlic powder

(optional), extra virgin olive oil, salt, and pepper all together to have a juicy sauce.

2. Marinate your trout with the sauce. For better taste, you may need to let it rest at room temperature for 30 minutes.
3. Preheat your oven to 375 °F.
4. Choose a long foil sheet, put trout in your foil sheet and close it. Let it cook for about 25 minutes until inside cooks well.
5. Enjoy!

<u>Cooking Tips:</u>

- Check your trout until inside cooked well. You may need more minutes for perfection.
- This dish can be served with potatoes or steamed white rice.
- You can substitute orange with lemon juice if you like to try other great flavors.

<u>Fructose Intolerance-related Tips:</u>

- Do not use black pepper and garlic powder if you are experiencing a flare-up.

Nutrition Facts	
Servings: 4	
Amount per serving	
Calories	**391**
	% Daily Value*
Total Fat 16.9g	22%
Saturated Fat 2.8g	14%
Cholesterol 115mg	38%
Sodium 105mg	5%
Total Carbohydrate 16.5g	6%
Dietary Fiber 3.4g	12%
Total Sugars 13g	
Protein 42.6g	
Vitamin D 0mcg	0%
Calcium 141mg	11%
Iron 3mg	18%
Potassium 980mg	21%

CHICKEN AND SHRIMP TERIYAKI

A lovely Edo-style mix of chicken and shrimp with healthy ingredients for people with fructose intolerance.

- Prep Time: 5 minutes
- Cook Time: 20 minutes
- Total Time: 25 minutes
- Serving: 4

<u>Ingredients</u>

- 2 lbs (~1 kg) organic chicken breast, chopped in cubes
- 24 shrimps, peeled and deveined
- 1 tablespoon ginseng powder, divided
- 2 tablespoons extra virgin olive oil
- ½ teaspoon turmeric
- ⅓ cup gluten-free and sodium-reduced soy sauce (optional)
- ⅓ cup of cold water
- 3 teaspoons arrowroot powder
- ¼ cup brown sugar
- Salt & pepper to taste

<u>Instructions</u>

1. In a medium bowl, whisk ginseng powder, one tablespoon of olive oil, soy sauce, arrowroot powder, or brown sugar, water, salt, and pepper to make a juicy teriyaki sauce.
2. Let Teriyaki sauce rest in the fridge for 5 minutes.
3. In a large pan, add one tablespoon of olive oil and cook chicken over medium heat until golden brown both sides.

4. Add your sauce and shrimp to the pan. Stir and mix for 5 minutes until thickened.
5. Enjoy!

<u>Cooking Tips:</u>

- You can serve this dish with steamed white rice or rice noodles.

<u>Fructose Intolerance-related Tips:</u>

- Do not use black pepper if you are experiencing a severe flare-up.
- Use soy sauce only if you can tolerate it.

Nutrition Facts

Servings: 4

Amount per serving	
Calories	**553**

	% Daily Value*
Total Fat 15.1g	19%
Saturated Fat 1.7g	9%
Cholesterol 423mg	141%
Sodium 1639mg	71%
Total Carbohydrate 20g	7%
Dietary Fiber 0.4g	1%
Total Sugars 12.1g	
Protein 79.6g	
Vitamin D 0mcg	1%
Calcium 151mg	12%
Iron 2mg	12%
Potassium 1175mg	25%

LEMON SHRIMP WITH WHITE RICE

Lemon Shrimp with steamed white rice is very easy to make and a healthy dish you can have in your weekly diet.

- Prep Time: 5 minutes
- Cook Time: 20 minutes
- Total Time: 25 minutes
- Serving: 4

<u>Ingredients</u>

- 24 shrimps, peeled and deveined
- 2 tablespoons extra virgin olive oil, divided
- ½ teaspoon turmeric powder
- 4 tablespoons lemon juice
- 3 cups of white rice
- 1 teaspoon salt & pepper
- 1 teaspoon garlic powder (optional)

Instructions

1. In a small bowl, whisk lemon juice, garlic powder (optional), one tablespoon of olive oil, turmeric powder, salt, and pepper to make a sauce.
2. Cook your rice according to its package instructions.
3. Add one tablespoon of high-quality extra virgin olive oil in a pan and cook shrimp over medium heat for 5-7 minutes.
4. Add your sauce into the pan. Stir and mix well for 5 minutes.
5. Enjoy!

Cooking Tips:

- You can serve the lemon shrimp with rice noodles instead of white rice.

Fructose Intolerance-related Tips:

- Do not use black pepper and garlic powder if you are experiencing a severe flare-up.

Nutrition Facts

Servings: 4

Amount per serving

Calories **729**

% Daily Value*

Total Fat 10.3g	13%
Saturated Fat 2.1g	10%
Cholesterol 278mg	93%
Sodium 332mg	14%
Total Carbohydrate 113.8g	41%
Dietary Fiber 2.1g	7%
Total Sugars 0.5g	
Protein 40.2g	
Vitamin D 0mcg	0%
Calcium 162mg	12%
Iron 7mg	37%
Potassium 416mg	9%

PRAWN LINGUINE

Are you looking for an Italian seafood linguine recipe for people with fructose intolerance? You have to try this delicious main course.

- Prep Time: 5 minutes
- Cook Time: 20 minutes
- Total Time: 25 minutes
- Serving: 4

Ingredients:

- 1 lb (~500 gr) prawns, peeled and deveined
- 1 lb (~500 gr) cooked gluten-free linguine
- 2 tablespoons extra virgin olive oil, divided
- 4 tablespoons brown sugar
- ½ cup carrot
- ½ cup of water
- Salt and black pepper to taste
- ¼ cup green onion (only if tolerated)
- 1 teaspoon garlic powder (optional)

Instructions

1. Whisk brown sugar, garlic powder (optional), one tablespoon of olive oil, carrot, green onion, pepper, and salt in a proper bowl to make a sauce.
2. Cook your linguini according to its package instructions.
3. Add one tablespoon of high-quality extra virgin olive oil in a medium-size pan and cook prawns over medium heat for 5-7 minutes.
4. Add your sauce into the pan. Stir and mix well for 5 minutes until sauce gets thick.
5. Add pasta to your sauce and mix all well. Enjoy!

<u>Cooking Tips:</u>

- You can serve the prawn linguine with rice noodles or any other kinds of gluten-free pasta instead of gluten-free linguini.

<u>Fructose Intolerance-related Tips:</u>

- Do not use black pepper, green onion, and garlic powder if you are experiencing a severe flare-up.

Nutrition Facts
Servings: 4

Amount per serving

Calories	592
	% Daily Value*
Total Fat 11.5g	15%
Saturated Fat 2g	10%
Cholesterol 322mg	107%
Sodium 317mg	14%
Total Carbohydrate 82.7g	30%
Dietary Fiber 0.5g	2%
Total Sugars 18g	
Protein 38.9g	
Vitamin D 0mcg	0%
Calcium 128mg	10%
Iron 4mg	24%
Potassium 461mg	10%

DESSERTS

PINEAPPLE CAKE SUNDAES

A delicious dessert with pineapple, cinnamon, and ice cream. Substantially modified to be consumed by people with fructose intolerance.

- Prep Time: 15 minutes
- Total Time: 15 minutes
- Serving: 4

Ingredients

- 2 tablespoons extra virgin olive oil
- ¼ cup white sugar
- 1 cup pineapple, chopped
- 1-pint lactose-free vanilla ice cream or sorbet
- 1½ cup vanilla loaf pound cake (GF)
- 1 tablespoon brown sugar
- ¼ teaspoon cinnamon powder

Instructions

- In a medium skillet, heat extra virgin olive oil over medium heat. Add sugar, cinnamon, and brown sugar. Stir well until brown with a soft texture.
- Add pineapple and let it cook for two-three more minutes. Remove from heat.
- Preheat oven to 375 °F. Bake your GF cake for about 8-10 minutes until toasted.
- Crumble vanilla loaf pound cake and place it on top of ice cream scoops (or sorbets).
- Add pineapple sauce. Serve and enjoy!

Cooking Tips:

- You can mix the pineapple sauce with any cold lactose-free plain or vanilla yogurt instead of ice cream.

Nutrition Facts	
Servings: 4	
Amount per serving	
Calories	**213**
	% Daily Value*
Total Fat 10.8g	14%
Saturated Fat 2.6g	13%
Cholesterol 12mg	4%
Sodium 54mg	2%
Total Carbohydrate 29g	11%
Dietary Fiber 0.7g	3%
Total Sugars 23.5g	
Protein 1.4g	
Vitamin D 0mcg	0%
Calcium 41mg	3%
Iron 1mg	3%
Potassium 78mg	2%

BANANA-GINSENG SUNDAES

This summer sundae is based on a great combination of banana, ginseng, and ice cream.

- Prep Time: 20 minutes
- Total Time: 20 minutes
- Serving: 4

<u>Ingredients</u>

- 2 bananas, peeled and sliced
- 2 tablespoons extra virgin olive oil
- 2 tablespoons brown sugar
- 6 tablespoons organic no added sugar, pineapple juice
- ½ teaspoon cornstarch
- 2 cup lactose-free vanilla ice cream or sorbet
- ¼ teaspoon freshly grated ginseng

<u>Instructions</u>

- In a large skillet, heat extra virgin olive oil over medium heat. Add banana and ginseng and cook for three minutes until tender. Add sugar and stir well for 1-2 minutes.
- In a bowl, mix cornstarch and pineapple juice and pour the mix into the skillet. Cook all mix until thickened.
- Cool for 2-4 minutes.
- Scoop your ice cream or sorbet in a proper dessert plate. Pour your mix on top.
- Serve and enjoy!

<u>Cooking Tips:</u>

- You can mix the ginseng sauce with any cold lactose-free plain or vanilla yogurts instead of ice cream.

<u>Fructose Intolerance-related Tips:</u>

- If you cannot tolerate cornstarch well, use rice flour.

Nutrition Facts

Servings: 4

Amount per serving	
Calories	**212**
	% Daily Value*
Total Fat 10.7g	14%
Saturated Fat 3.3g	16%
Cholesterol 10mg	3%
Sodium 20mg	1%
Total Carbohydrate 29.7g	11%
Dietary Fiber 2.7g	10%
Total Sugars 25.2g	
Protein 1.3g	
Vitamin D 0mcg	0%
Calcium 46mg	4%
Iron 1mg	3%
Potassium 151mg	3%

Banana Lemon Trifle

If you want to try a different delicious dessert, you have to make Banana Lemon Trifle.

- Prep Time: 10 minutes
- Total Time: 20 minutes
- Serving: 6

Ingredients

- 4 packs instant gluten-free vanilla pudding
- 3 packs gluten-free shortbread cookies
- ½ cup low fat lactose-free milk or almond milk
- 3 bananas, sliced
- 1 tablespoon lemon juice
- Lemon zest
- 4-5 fresh mint leaves

Instructions

- In a large bowl, prepare vanilla pudding according to package instructions. Then mix pudding with lemon juice, lemon zest, and almond milk.
- Top the bowl with shredded shortbread cookies and sliced banana. Garnish with mint leaves.

Cooking Tips:

- You can top the bowl with cinnamon powder as well.

Fructose Intolerance-related Tips:

- Make sure you can tolerate mint leaves. Otherwise, do not use it.

Nutrition Facts

Servings: 6

Amount per serving

Calories 481

	% Daily Value*
Total Fat 11.2g	14%
Saturated Fat 6.4g	32%
Cholesterol 28mg	9%
Sodium 1033mg	45%
Total Carbohydrate 94.1g	34%
Dietary Fiber 2.6g	9%
Total Sugars 74.3g	
Protein 2.4g	
Vitamin D 0mcg	0%
Calcium 21mg	2%
Iron 1mg	4%
Potassium 253mg	5%

GINSENG FRUIT SHERBET

Try tasting new! A fantastic sherbet made from ginseng, orange, and pineapple.

- Prep Time: 5 minutes
- Freeze Time: 20 minutes
- Total Time: 25 minutes
- Serving: 4

Ingredients

- 1 cup pineapple, diced
- 5 tablespoons orange marmalade/jam
- 2 cups orange, lemon, pineapple or lime sherbet
- 1 tablespoon freshly grated ginseng
- 1 table spoon brown sugar
- ¼ teaspoon vanilla

Instructions

- In a large bowl, mix well all ingredients together.
- Chill the bowl for 15 minutes in your freezer.
- Remove from the freezer and refrigerate for five more minutes.

- Remove from the fridge. Stir the mix a bit, and enjoy it!

<u>Making Tips:</u>

- Add one more tablespoon of freshly grated ginseng or ginseng powder if you want to have a ginseng flavor more.
- Try to find sugar-free marmalade or jam. If you cannot find it, you can make it fast at home by mixing orange, orange zest, and brown sugar. Then, refrigerate it for an hour.

<u>Fructose Intolerance-related Tips:</u>

- Orange can irritate the gut in some people with fructose intolerance. Make sure you can tolerate orange. If you cannot, make a pineapple version by using a pineapple- brown sugar mixture instead of orange marmalade.

Nutrition Facts

Servings: 4

Amount per serving

Calories	147
	% Daily Value*
Total Fat 0.6g	1%
Saturated Fat 0.3g	1%
Cholesterol 3mg	1%
Sodium 23mg	1%
Total Carbohydrate 36.6g	13%
Dietary Fiber 0.9g	3%
Total Sugars 30.1g	
Protein 0.9g	
Vitamin D 0mcg	0%
Calcium 27mg	2%
Iron 0mg	2%
Potassium 73mg	2%

PINEAPPLE QUESADILLAS

If you can tolerate tortilla or can find gluten-free tortillas, then this dessert is an excellent option for you to make. It perfectly comes with ice cream on top.

- Prep Time: 10 minutes
- Cook Time: 10 minutes
- Total Time: 20 minutes
- Serving: 4-6

Ingredients

- 4 pieces of gluten-free tortillas
- 1 cup old cheddar cheese (lactose-free), shredded
- 1 tablespoon extra virgin olive oil
- ½ pineapple, sliced
- 2 tablespoons brown sugar
- 4 tablespoons lactose-free ice cream or sorbet

Instructions

1. Preheat oven to 375 °F.
2. Place your tortillas on a proper baking sheet. Sprinkle extra virgin olive oil, and top with cheese, brown sugar, and thinly sliced pineapples on half of each tortilla.
3. Wrap tortilla by folding the other half towards the half with mixture.
4. Bake quesadillas for about 7-10 minutes until golden.
5. Scoop ice cream or sorbet and top it with your mix. Enjoy!

Fructose Intolerance-related Tips:

- When in a flare-up, do not have ice cream with your pineapple quesadillas.

Nutrition Facts	
Servings: 6	
Amount per serving	
Calories	**323**
	% Daily Value*
Total Fat 19.4g	25%
Saturated Fat 7.7g	38%
Cholesterol 35mg	12%
Sodium 155mg	7%
Total Carbohydrate 31.2g	11%
Dietary Fiber 7.1g	25%
Total Sugars 20g	
Protein 13.4g	
Vitamin D 0mcg	0%
Calcium 56mg	4%
Iron 0mg	2%
Potassium 84mg	2%

MIDDLE-EASTERN RICE PUDDING

Rice pudding is a well-known dessert everywhere. Try a luxurious taste of new rice pudding for people with fructose intolerance!

- Prep Time: 10 minutes
- Cook Time: 30 minutes
- Total Time: 40 minutes
- Serving: 4-6

Ingredients

- 1 cup white rice
- 2 cups lactose-free milk
- ¾ cup brown sugar
- ½ teaspoon grated cinnamon
- 2 tablespoons extra virgin olive oil
- 2 cups of water
- ½ cup rosewater (optional)

Instructions

1. In a medium pot, put rice and add boiling water. Let the rice boil over low heat until all water evaporates.

2. Add milk until boiled. Stir consistently.
3. Add brown sugar and rose water (optional) and stir for 3-5 more minutes. Add cinnamon powder on top.
4. Serve warm or cold. Enjoy!

<u>Cooking Tips:</u>

- It is highly recommended to use rosewater in this rice pudding to experience a luxurious taste!
- If you want to have a delicious yellow rice pudding, add ⅓ teaspoon grounded saffron.

Nutrition Facts

Servings: 6

Amount per serving

Calories — **290**

	% Daily Value*
Total Fat 5.7g	7%
Saturated Fat 1.3g	6%
Cholesterol 4mg	1%
Sodium 41mg	2%
Total Carbohydrate 55.3g	20%
Dietary Fiber 0.5g	2%
Total Sugars 27.7g	
Protein 5g	
Vitamin D 42mcg	211%
Calcium 134mg	10%
Iron 2mg	10%
Potassium 239mg	5%

GLUTEN-FREE STRAWBERRY PIE

This homemade gluten-free strawberry made with almond flour can satisfy you and your gut!

- Prep Time: 30 minutes
- Cook Time: 55 minutes
- Total Time: 85 minutes
- Serving: 6

<u>Ingredients</u>

- 1¾ cups almond flour, grounded

- ¼ cup tapioca flour+2 tablespoons tapioca flour
- 6 tablespoons extra virgin olive oil
- ½ large egg whisked
- 1 cup rolled oats or gluten-free oats
- 1 cup brown sugar
- 1 teaspoon cinnamon powder
- ½ teaspoon ground ginseng
- 20 strawberries, sliced
- 1 tablespoon lemon juice
- 1 tablespoon vanilla extract
- Salt, to taste

Instructions

1. In a large bowl, mix almond and tapioca flour rolled oats and olive oil.
2. In a bowl, whisk egg a bit and adds ½ of an egg into the dough. Mix well to form a soft-ball. If the texture is not good, add 1 or 2 teaspoons of the whisked egg to the dough.
3. Put your dough on a parchment paper. Fridge the dough for an hour (Recommended keeping it in a fridge overnight).
4. Remove from the fridge. With a rolling pin, make a 10-12 inch disk. Then, gently move your dough disk to the pie plate. Return into its shape again if any part falls apart or breaks.
5. Crimp the edges with your fingertips. Make small holes in all parts of your dough.
6. In a large bowl, mix thinly sliced strawberries with lemon juice, vanilla extract, sugar, ginseng, and salt.
7. Cover your crust with the mix altogether.
8. Preheat oven to 400 °F.

9. Cover crust edges with a pie shield to avoid burning fast.

10. Bake for 15-20 minutes. Reduce heat to 350°F and let it bake for 40 minutes.

11. Remove from the oven. Cool down. Slice it and serve.

<u>Cooking Tips:</u>

- Cover the pie with aluminum foil if you see the toppings are getting brown so fast.

Nutrition Facts
Servings: 6

Amount per serving

Calories	380
	% Daily Value*
Total Fat 23.4g	30%
Saturated Fat 2.8g	14%
Cholesterol 14mg	5%
Sodium 18mg	1%
Total Carbohydrate 40.5g	15%
Dietary Fiber 6.1g	22%
Total Sugars 16.5g	
Protein 5.3g	
Vitamin D 1mcg	6%
Calcium 43mg	3%
Iron 2mg	10%
Potassium 299mg	6%

PUMPKIN PIE

Enjoy cooking a traditional pumpkin pie recipe for people with fructose intolerance!

- Prep Time: 15 minutes
- Cook Time: 55 minutes
- Total Time: 70 minutes
- Serving: 4-6

<u>Ingredients</u>

- 2 cups pumpkin, peeled
- 1 ready pie crust, gluten-free (9-inch)

- 2 organic, free-range eggs
- 1.5 cups unsweetened condensed milk
- ½ teaspoon freshly grated ginseng
- ½ teaspoon cinnamon powder
- ½ teaspoon salt

Instructions

1. Preheat oven to 400°F.
2. Blend the pumpkin with all other ingredients in a blender or whisk all ingredients in a large bowl.
3. Pour the mix in a ready crust and bake for 15 minutes.
4. Reduce heat to 350 °F and let it bake for 35-40 minutes. You can insert a fork into it. The fork has to come out very clean, showing that it perfectly cooked.
5. Serve and enjoy!

Cooking Tips:

- Cover the pie with aluminum foil if you see the toppings are getting brown so fast.

Nutrition Facts

Servings: 6

Amount per serving	
Calories	**403**
	% Daily Value*
Total Fat 15.3g	20%
Saturated Fat 5.8g	29%
Cholesterol 81mg	27%
Sodium 258mg	11%
Total Carbohydrate 58.9g	21%
Dietary Fiber 2.6g	9%
Total Sugars 45.3g	
Protein 9.7g	
Vitamin D 5mcg	26%
Calcium 251mg	19%
Iron 2mg	11%
Potassium 497mg	11%

FRUIT DESSERT

A fresh cold fruit mix as a healthy dessert choice for people with fructose intolerance.

- Prep Time: 20 minutes
- Total Time: 20 minutes
- Serving: 4

<u>Ingredients</u>

- 2 cups pineapple, cubed
- 2 cups cantaloupe, cubed
- 1 tablespoon brown sugar
- 3 tablespoons lime juice
- 1 cup papaya, cubed

<u>Instructions</u>

1. In a large bowl, mix all ingredients.
2. Serve cold. Enjoy!

<u>Cooking Tips:</u>

- You can change the fruits in your fruit dessert as you wish, but make sure you can tolerate those fruits and always peel them off.
- You can mix your fruits with lactose-free plain yogurt, as well.

Nutrition Facts	
Servings: 4	
Amount per serving	
Calories	**132**
	% Daily Value*
Total Fat 0.5g	1%
Saturated Fat 0.1g	1%
Cholesterol 0mg	0%
Sodium 33mg	1%
Total Carbohydrate 34g	12%
Dietary Fiber 3.3g	12%
Total Sugars 27.3g	
Protein 1.8g	
Vitamin D 0mcg	0%
Calcium 36mg	3%
Iron 1mg	4%
Potassium 594mg	13%

Avocado Blueberry Popsicle

Homemade popsicles are great desserts for people with fructose intolerance. It is very easy to make popsicles at home. You need to try this recipe as an example:

- Prep Time: 10 minutes
- Freeze Time: 90 minutes
- Total Time: 100 minutes
- Serving: 4

Ingredients

- 2 avocados, peeled
- 1 cup blueberries

Instructions

1. Blend well blueberries and avocados in a blender or food processor.
2. Fill up your Popsicle cups. Insert popsicle sticks and freeze.
3. Run the outside of the cup under hot water to remove the popsicles when you want to eat it.

<u>Cooking Tips:</u>

- You can change the fruit(s) in your popsicle as you wish, but make sure you can tolerate those fruits and always peel them off.

Nutrition Facts

Servings: 4

Amount per serving

Calories   **245**

	% Daily Value*
Total Fat 19.7g	25%
Saturated Fat 4.1g	21%
Cholesterol 0mg	0%
Sodium 7mg	0%
Total Carbohydrate 19.2g	7%
Dietary Fiber 8.9g	32%
Total Sugars 7.3g	
Protein 2.2g	
Vitamin D 0mcg	0%
Calcium 18mg	1%
Iron 1mg	4%
Potassium 568mg	12%

LEMON SORBET

Try a Paleo-kind refreshing sorbet with great combinations of lemon juice and brown sugar.

- Prep Time: 10 minutes
- Make Time: 120 minutes
- Total Time: 130 minutes
- Serving: 4

<u>Ingredients</u>

- 1 cup fresh lemon juice
- 2 tablespoons lemon zest
- 2 cups of water
- ½ cup brown sugar
- 1 cup light cream

<u>Instructions</u>

1. In a medium pot, mix your brown sugar, lemon zest, and water until the brown sugar dissolves and gets warm.
2. Add lemon juice or squeeze a lemon to the pot. Stir a bit.
3. Pour your sorbet mixture into a metal pan or pot or an ice cream maker.
4. Freeze for 2 hours. Scrape the sorbet with a spoon or fork every 15 minutes.
5. Enjoy!

<u>Cooking Tips:</u>

- You can change the fruit(s) in your sorbet as you wish, but make sure you can tolerate those fruits and always peel them off.

<u>Fructose Intolerance-related Tips:</u>

- Make sure you can tolerate light cream. Instead, you can use almond milk. Be aware that it may need more freezing time if you use almond milk.

Nutrition Facts

Servings: 4

Amount per serving	
Calories	**234**
	% Daily Value*
Total Fat 9.8g	13%
Saturated Fat 6.3g	31%
Cholesterol 33mg	11%
Sodium 24mg	1%
Total Carbohydrate 37.7g	14%
Dietary Fiber 0.5g	2%
Total Sugars 36.3g	
Protein 1.3g	
Vitamin D 0mcg	0%
Calcium 29mg	2%
Iron 0mg	1%
Potassium 136mg	3%

PINEAPPLE ICE CREAM

This dairy-free pineapple ice cream is very easy to make. It is healthy and a tasty dessert choice for people with fructose intolerance.

- Prep Time: 15 minutes
- Cook Time: 30 minutes
- Total Time: 45 minutes
- Serving: 6

<u>Ingredients</u>

- 1¾ cup almond milk
- 2 cups pineapple, sliced
- ¼ cup brown sugar
- ½ teaspoon vanilla extract

<u>Instructions</u>

1. Perfectly chill your almond milk in a fridge before you make this ice cream.
2. Blend milk, pineapples, brown sugar, and vanilla extract in a blender until perfectly smooth.
3. Pour your sorbet mixture into a metal container, pot, or an ice cream maker. If you use an ice cream maker, it takes about 30 minutes, but if you use a metal container, you may need to freeze it for 90-120 minutes.
4. Serve cold and enjoy it!

<u>Cooking Tips:</u>

- You can change the fruits in your ice cream as you desire, but make sure you can tolerate those fruits and always peel them off.

Nutrition Facts	
Servings: 6	
Amount per serving	
Calories	**272**
	% Daily Value*
Total Fat 17.1g	22%
Saturated Fat 14.9g	75%
Cholesterol 0mg	0%
Sodium 12mg	1%
Total Carbohydrate 32.3g	12%
Dietary Fiber 3.4g	12%
Total Sugars 29.3g	
Protein 2.6g	
Vitamin D 0mcg	0%
Calcium 24mg	2%
Iron 1mg	8%
Potassium 380mg	8%

SWEET POTATO PIE

If you want to make a pie with potato as a dessert, you can follow the recipe of sweet potato pie.

- Prep Time: 30 minutes
- Cook Time: 50 minutes
- Total Time: 80 minutes
- Serving: 4-6

<u>Ingredients</u>

- 2 medium sweet potatoes, peeled and cubed
- ¾ cup unsweetened condensed milk
- 1 deep-dish pie shell, uncooked (or gluten-free pastry shell)
- 2 tablespoons extra virgin olive oil
- ½ cup brown sugar
- 2 large organic, free-range eggs
- 1 teaspoon vanilla extract
- ½ teaspoon cinnamon powder
- ½ teaspoon ground nutmeg
- ¼ teaspoon salt

<u>Instructions</u>

1. In a large pot, boil sweet potatoes by boiling water over medium heat.
2. Drain and mash potatoes by fork or blender.
3. Preheat oven to 400°F.
4. Mix mashed sweet potatoes with extra virgin olive oil, sugar, eggs, cinnamon, vanilla, nutmeg, and salt perfectly in a large bowl.
5. Pour the mix into a ready pie shell. Bake it for 20 minutes. Then, reduce heat around 350 °F and bake for 30-35 more minutes.
6. Serve warm or cold. Enjoy!

<u>Cooking Tips:</u>

-   Cover the pie shell with aluminum foil if you see the toppings are getting brown so fast.

<u>Fructose Intolerance-related Tips:</u>

-   Make sure you can tolerate nutmeg. If you cannot, remove it from the ingredients.

Nutrition Facts

Servings: 6

Amount per serving	
Calories	**392**
	% Daily Value*
Total Fat 16.6g	21%
Saturated Fat 3.4g	17%
Cholesterol 75mg	25%
Sodium 74mg	3%
Total Carbohydrate 44.8g	16%
Dietary Fiber 1.1g	4%
Total Sugars 37.9g	
Protein 6.5g	
Vitamin D 6mcg	29%
Calcium 122mg	9%
Iron 1mg	3%
Potassium 370mg	8%

WHITE PANNA COTTA

A dairy-free, easy to make panna cotta for people with fructose intolerance that comes with a lovely creamy taste of almond milk.

- Prep Time: 10 minutes
- Chill time: 120 minutes
- Total Time: 130 minutes
- Serving: 4

<u>Ingredients</u>

- 1¾ cup almond milk
- ⅓ cup brown sugar
- 2 teaspoons gelatin, grass-fed
- 1 teaspoon vanilla extract

<u>Instructions</u>

1. In a medium pan, heat almond milk and add gelatin. Stir until gelatin powder melts.
2. Add vanilla. Stir and let the mix get warmer for 3-5 minutes over medium heat until gelatin fully dissolved. Be aware that you should not boil the milk.
3. Remove from pan and add brown sugar. Stir well.
4. Fill some small cups with the mixture and fridge it for 3-4 hours.
5. To remove Panna Cotta easily, put small cups in a hot water bowl for 2 minutes. Then, you can flip Panna Cottas on your dessert plates. Enjoy!

<u>Cooking Tips:</u>

- For having a fruity Panna Cotta, you can add poached and peeled tolerable fruit cubes in your mixture, as well.

- Alternatively, you can garnish your panna cotta with fruits you can tolerate.

Nutrition Facts
Servings: 4

Amount per serving

Calories	325
	% Daily Value*
Total Fat 25.1g	32%
Saturated Fat 22.2g	111%
Cholesterol 0mg	0%
Sodium 25mg	1%
Total Carbohydrate 23.6g	9%
Dietary Fiber 2.3g	8%
Total Sugars 19.3g	
Protein 5.4g	
Vitamin D 0mcg	0%
Calcium 36mg	3%
Iron 2mg	12%
Potassium 332mg	7%

COCKTAILS AND SHAKES

BANANA MILKSHAKE

Enjoy tasting a traditional milkshake with banana.

- Prep Time: 5 minutes
- Serving: 1

Ingredients

- 1 banana
- 1 cup unsweetened almond or lactose-free milk
- 2 tablespoons brown sugar

Instructions

- Blend all the above ingredients until smooth. Pour into a large glass. Enjoy!

Nutrition Facts	
Servings: 1	
Amount per serving	
Calories	**145**
	% Daily Value*
Total Fat 3.9g	5%
Saturated Fat 0.4g	2%
Cholesterol 0mg	0%
Sodium 181mg	8%
Total Carbohydrate 29g	11%
Dietary Fiber 4.1g	15%
Total Sugars 14.4g	
Protein 2.3g	
Vitamin D 1mcg	7%
Calcium 306mg	24%
Iron 1mg	6%
Potassium 612mg	13%

COOLER DRINK

Enjoy tasting a great drink that makes you really cool!

- Prep Time: 5 minutes
- Serving: 1

Ingredients

- 2 cucumbers, peeled
- 10 mint leaves
- 1 cup lemon juice
- 1 cup of water
- Ice cubes

Instructions

- Blend all ingredients in a blender and then blend until smooth. Pour into a large glass. Enjoy!

Cooking Tips:

- You can add one teaspoon of freshly grated ginseng to the drink as well.

Nutrition Facts	
Servings: 1	
Amount per serving	
Calories	**193**
	% Daily Value*
Total Fat 3.3g	4%
Saturated Fat 2.4g	12%
Cholesterol 0mg	0%
Sodium 91mg	4%
Total Carbohydrate 35.4g	13%
Dietary Fiber 10.8g	39%
Total Sugars 15.2g	
Protein 9.2g	
Vitamin D 0mcg	0%
Calcium 312mg	24%
Iron 14mg	76%
Potassium 1646mg	35%

STRAWBERRY-BANANA SMOOTHIE

A great smoothie with strawberry and banana!

- Prep Time: 5 minutes
- Serving: 1-2

Ingredients

- 1 cup strawberry, diced
- 1 banana, diced
- 1 cup lactose-free milk or almond milk
- ½ teaspoon brown sugar

Instructions

- Blend all ingredients in a blender and then blend until smooth. Pour into a large glass. Enjoy!

Cooking Tips:

- You can use plain lactose-free yogurt or banana lactose-free yogurt instead of milk for having a thick texture.
- You can add ½ cup of papaya to the mix as well.

Nutrition Facts	
Servings: 2	
Amount per serving	
Calories	**218**
	% Daily Value*
Total Fat 3.4g	4%
Saturated Fat 1.7g	9%
Cholesterol 11mg	4%
Sodium 62mg	3%
Total Carbohydrate 44.7g	16%
Dietary Fiber 4.2g	15%
Total Sugars 30.2g	
Protein 6.3g	
Vitamin D 50mcg	250%
Calcium 171mg	13%
Iron 0mg	2%
Potassium 703mg	15%

AVOCADO SMOOTHIE

A great healthy drink for people with fructose intolerance with healthy fats. If you like, you can add protein powder in the smoothie.

- Prep Time: 5 minutes
- Serving: 1-2

Ingredients

- 1 avocado
- 1 banana
- 1 cup lactose-free milk or unsweetened almond milk
- 2 tablespoons brown sugar

Instructions

- Blend all ingredients in a blender and then blend until smooth. Pour into a large glass. Enjoy!

Nutrition Facts

Servings: 2

Amount per serving

Calories   **375**

	% Daily Value*
Total Fat 22.3g	29%
Saturated Fat 5.7g	29%
Cholesterol 10mg	3%
Sodium 71mg	3%
Total Carbohydrate 42g	15%
Dietary Fiber 8.3g	30%
Total Sugars 25.6g	
Protein 6.6g	
Vitamin D 0mcg	0%
Calcium 178mg	14%
Iron 1mg	6%
Potassium 739mg	16%

Banana-Cinnamon Smoothie

A classical thick smoothie to enjoy!

- Prep Time: 5 minutes
- Serving: 1

<u>Ingredients</u>

- 1 banana
- 1 cup lactose-free vanilla yogurt
- 2 tablespoons brown sugar
- 1 teaspoon cinnamon
- ⅓ cup of ice

<u>Instructions</u>

- Blend all ingredients in a blender and then blend until smooth. Pour into a large glass. Enjoy!

<u>Cooking Tips:</u>

- Plain yogurt can also be used instead of vanilla yogurt.

Nutrition Facts	
Servings: 1	
Amount per serving	
Calories	**320**
	% Daily Value*
Total Fat 3.5g	4%
Saturated Fat 2.6g	13%
Cholesterol 15mg	5%
Sodium 174mg	8%
Total Carbohydrate 55g	20%
Dietary Fiber 4.3g	15%
Total Sugars 39.7g	
Protein 15.3g	
Vitamin D 0mcg	0%
Calcium 486mg	37%
Iron 1mg	5%
Potassium 1033mg	22%

PINEAPPLE-BLUEBERRY-BLACKBERRY SMOOTHIE

A fabulous smoothie with three different fruits to enjoy!

- Prep Time: 5 minutes
- Serving: 1-2

Ingredients

- ½ cup blueberry, diced
- ½ blackberry, diced
- 1 cup pineapple, diced
- 1 cup lactose-free plain yogurt
- ½ cup of ice
- 1 tablespoon brown sugar

Instructions

- Blend all ingredients in a blender and then blend until smooth. Pour into a large glass. Enjoy!

Fructose Intolerance-related Tips:

- You can add papaya to the mix as well.

PINEAPPLE-GINSENG SMOOTHIE

A ginseng-based smoothie with a fantastic taste!

- Prep Time: 5 minutes
- Serving: 1

Ingredients

- 1 cup pineapple, diced
- 1 cup lactose-free milk or unsweetened almond milk
- 1 tablespoon fresh grated ginseng
- 1 tablespoon brown sugar

Instructions

- Blend all ingredients in a blender and then blend until smooth. Pour into a large glass. Enjoy!

Nutrition Facts

Servings: 1

Amount per serving	
Calories	**208**
	% Daily Value*
Total Fat 5.7g	7%
Saturated Fat 3.1g	16%
Cholesterol 20mg	7%
Sodium 127mg	6%
Total Carbohydrate 30.8g	11%
Dietary Fiber 3g	11%
Total Sugars 26.2g	
Protein 9.9g	
Vitamin D 0mcg	0%
Calcium 306mg	24%
Iron 1mg	5%
Potassium 358mg	8%

POMEGRANATE-ANGELICA SMOOTHIE

Enjoy a healthy smoothie with a fantastic sour taste!

- Prep Time: 5 minutes
- Serving: 1-2

Ingredients

- 1 cup pomegranate juice
- ½ cup plain lactose-free yogurt
- 1 tablespoon Angelica root powder (optional)
- 1 teaspoon salt

Instructions

- Blend all ingredients in a blender and then blend until smooth. Pour into a large glass. Enjoy!

Cooking Tips:

- You can use one tablespoon of maple syrup for giving sweetness to the smoothie if you can tolerate it.

Nutrition Facts

Servings: 1

Amount per serving

Calories	237

	% Daily Value*
Total Fat 1.5g	2%
Saturated Fat 1.2g	6%
Cholesterol 7mg	2%
Sodium 2421mg	105%
Total Carbohydrate 45.6g	17%
Dietary Fiber 0g	0%
Total Sugars 40.6g	
Protein 7g	
Vitamin D 0mcg	0%
Calcium 246mg	19%
Iron 0mg	1%
Potassium 887mg	19%

BANANA-CINNAMON-GINSENG SMOOTHIE

A ginseng-based smoothie with a fantastic taste!

- Prep Time: 5 minutes
- Serving: 1-2

Ingredients

- 1 banana, diced
- 1 cup lactose-free milk or unsweetened almond milk
- 3 tablespoons lime juice
- 1 teaspoon cinnamon
- 1 tablespoon fresh grated ginseng
- 1 tablespoon brown sugar

Instructions

- Blend all ingredients in a blender and then blend until smooth. Pour into a large glass. Enjoy!

Cooking Tips:

- You can use one tablespoon of maple syrup in this recipe if you can tolerate it well.

Nutrition Facts	
Servings: 1	
Amount per serving	
Calories	**345**
	% Daily Value*
Total Fat 5.8g	7%
Saturated Fat 3.1g	16%
Cholesterol 20mg	7%
Sodium 131mg	6%
Total Carbohydrate 70.5g	26%
Dietary Fiber 6.4g	23%
Total Sugars 53.7g	
Protein 9.4g	
Vitamin D 0mcg	0%
Calcium 318mg	24%
Iron 2mg	10%
Potassium 399mg	8%

PINEAPPLE-PAPAYA SMOOTHIE

Enjoy a great combination of pineapple and papaya in a refreshing smoothie!

- Prep Time: 5-7 minutes
- Serving: 2

<u>Ingredients</u>

- 1 cup papaya, diced
- 1 cup pineapple chunks
- 1 cup almond or lactose-free milk
- 1 tablespoon brown sugar

<u>Instructions</u>

- Blend all ingredients in a blender and then blend until smooth. Pour into a large glass. Enjoy!

Nutrition Facts

Servings: 2

Amount per serving

Calories   **398**

	% Daily Value*
Total Fat 29g	37%
Saturated Fat 25.5g	127%
Cholesterol 0mg	0%
Sodium 20mg	1%
Total Carbohydrate 38.5g	14%
Dietary Fiber 5.1g	18%
Total Sugars 32g	
Protein 3.9g	
Vitamin D 0mcg	0%
Calcium 39mg	3%
Iron 2mg	13%
Potassium 550mg	12%

CANTALOUPE SMOOTHIE

Enjoy a great smoothie with cantaloupe!

- Prep Time: 5 minutes
- Serving: 1-2

Ingredients

- 1 cup cantaloupe, diced
- ½ cup vanilla lactose-free yogurt
- ½ cup of orange juice
- 1 tablespoon brown sugar, to taste
- 2 ice cubes

Instructions

- Blend all ingredients in a blender and then blend until smooth. Pour into a large glass. Enjoy!

Fructose Intolerance-related Tips:

- If orange juice irritates your gut, simply remove it from the recipe.

Nutrition Facts	
Servings: 1	
Amount per serving	
Calories	**260**
	% Daily Value*
Total Fat 2.1g	3%
Saturated Fat 1.4g	7%
Cholesterol 7mg	2%
Sodium 113mg	5%
Total Carbohydrate 51.6g	19%
Dietary Fiber 1.7g	6%
Total Sugars 48.5g	
Protein 9.2g	
Vitamin D 0mcg	0%
Calcium 241mg	19%
Iron 2mg	11%
Potassium 962mg	20%

CANTALOUPE-MIX SMOOTHIE

Enjoy a great mix of cantaloupe with papaya, lemon, and orange!

- Prep Time: 5-10 minutes
- Serving: 2

<u>Ingredients</u>

- 1 cup cantaloupe, diced
- ½ cup papaya, diced
- ½ cup almond milk or lactose-free cow milk
- ½ cup of orange juice
- 2 tablespoons lemon
- 1 tablespoon maple syrup, to taste
- 2 ice cubes

<u>Instructions</u>

- Blend the ingredients in a blender until smooth. Pour into a large glass. Enjoy!

<u>Cooking Tips:</u>

<u>Fructose Intolerance-related Tips:</u>

- If orange juice irritates your gut, remove it from the recipe.

Nutrition Facts	
Servings: 2	
Amount per serving	
Calories	**253**
	% Daily Value*
Total Fat 14.8g	19%
Saturated Fat 12.8g	64%
Cholesterol 0mg	0%
Sodium 23mg	1%
Total Carbohydrate 32.2g	12%
Dietary Fiber 3.2g	11%
Total Sugars 27.9g	
Protein 3g	
Vitamin D 0mcg	0%
Calcium 26mg	2%
Iron 2mg	12%
Potassium 583mg	12%

Avocado Smoothie

Have you tried the taste of avocado milk? Try this smoothie cold!

- Prep Time: 5-7 minutes
- Serving: 1

Ingredients

- 1 cup unsweetened almond or lactose-free milk
- ½ avocado
- ¼ teaspoon ground cinnamon
- ½ cup ice

Instructions

- Blend all ingredients in a blender. Blend the mix until smooth. Pour into a large glass. Enjoy!

Cooking Tips:

- You can use 1 tablespoon of maple syrup for sweetness if you can tolerate it.

Nutrition Facts	
Servings: 1	
Amount per serving	
Calories	**299**
	% Daily Value*
Total Fat 23.2g	30%
Saturated Fat 4.4g	22%
Cholesterol 0mg	0%
Sodium 189mg	8%
Total Carbohydrate 24.9g	9%
Dietary Fiber 9.5g	34%
Total Sugars 12.8g	
Protein 3.1g	
Vitamin D 1mcg	7%
Calcium 322mg	25%
Iron 2mg	8%
Potassium 771mg	16%

PINA COLADA SMOOTHIE

A classical gluten-free Mexican smoothie for your parties!

- Prep Time: 5 minutes
- Serving: 1

Ingredients

- 1 cup pineapple chunks
- ½ cup unsweetened almond milk or lactose-free milk
- 1 banana
- ½ teaspoon coconut extract, to taste
- 1 tablespoon maple syrup (optional)

Instructions

- Blend all ingredients in a blender and then blend until smooth and creamy. Pour into a large glass. Enjoy!

Fructose Intolerance-related Tips:

- Do not use coconut extract if you are experiencing a flare-up.

Nutrition Facts	
Servings: 1	
Amount per serving	
Calories	**348**
	% Daily Value*
Total Fat 9g	12%
Saturated Fat 6.2g	31%
Cholesterol 0mg	0%
Sodium 98mg	4%
Total Carbohydrate 70.2g	26%
Dietary Fiber 7.7g	28%
Total Sugars 49.4g	
Protein 3.4g	
Vitamin D 1mcg	3%
Calcium 179mg	14%
Iron 4mg	22%
Potassium 783mg	17%

SNACKS

DICED FRUITS

You can dice fresh fruits you can tolerate and use them between your daily main meals. Papaya, cantaloupe, and pineapple are some of the best fruits for people with fructose intolerance.

PLAIN YOGURT WITH POACHED FRUITS

Another great snack is mixing lactose-free plain/vanilla yogurt with fruits you can tolerate or peeled and poached fruits.

POACHED FRUIT COMPOTE

It is a great choice that can be consumed by people with fructose intolerance.

- Prep Time: 10 minutes
- Cook Time: 40 Minutes
- Total Time: 50 minutes
- Serving: 6

Ingredients

- 1 cup papaya, skin removed and thinly sliced
- 1 cup pineapple, pitted and skin removed
- 1 teaspoon cinnamon powder
- 1 cup brown sugar
- 1 teaspoon vanilla extract

Instructions

1. In a large pot, cook fruits in boiling water over medium heat until softened.
2. In a large bowl, mix well all ingredients (except fruits) together.
3. Pour the syrup over fruits and let the compote be thickened.
4. Pour compote into a jar. Serve hot or cold. Enjoy!

Cooking Tips:

- You can poach fruits with the skin and remove the skin after poaching and before adding syrup to it.
- Make sure you wash fruits thoroughly after peeling them off.
- If you can tolerate sugar and for better sweetness, you can use ½ cup of white sugar.

Fructose Intolerance-related Tips:

- Always make and consume poached fruits you can tolerate.

Nutrition Facts

Nutrition Facts	
Servings: 6	
Amount per serving	
Calories	**232**
	% Daily Value*
Total Fat 0.3g	0%
Saturated Fat 0g	0%
Cholesterol 0mg	0%
Sodium 3mg	0%
Total Carbohydrate 61.1g	22%
Dietary Fiber 2.5g	9%
Total Sugars 59.7g	
Protein 1.2g	
Vitamin D 0mcg	0%
Calcium 4mg	0%
Iron 1mg	4%
Potassium 260mg	6%

AVOCADO DIP

A modified avocado dip recipe is a great snack candidate for people with fructose intolerance.

- Prep Time: 5 minutes
- Cook Time: 0 minutes
- Total Time: 5 minutes
- Serving: 4-6

<u>Ingredients</u>

- 6 avocados, peeled
- ½ tablespoon extra virgin olive oil
- ¼ cup chopped fresh cilantro
- 2 tablespoons fresh lime juice
- 1 teaspoon fresh lemon juice
- ½ teaspoon salt

<u>Instructions</u>

1. In a large bowl, mash avocados with a fork.
2. Add extra virgin olive oil and other ingredients into it.
3. Enjoy!

<u>Cooking Tips:</u>

- You can serve guacamole with gluten-free tacos if you can tolerate it.
- If you can tolerate a few tomatoes and onions, cube them and then add them into your guacamole.

<u>Fructose Intolerance-related Tips:</u>

- Do not use fresh cilantro if you are experiencing a severe flare-up.

Nutrition Facts

Servings: 6

Amount per serving

Calories	422
	% Daily Value*
Total Fat 40.4g	52%
Saturated Fat 8.4g	42%
Cholesterol 0mg	0%
Sodium 207mg	9%
Total Carbohydrate 18g	7%
Dietary Fiber 13.5g	48%
Total Sugars 1.2g	
Protein 3.9g	
Vitamin D 0mcg	0%
Calcium 26mg	2%
Iron 1mg	7%
Potassium 988mg	21%

HOMEMADE HUMMUS

A healthy and tasty middle-eastern snack. An excellent option for vegetarians and people with fructose intolerance during the remission period.

- Prep Time: 5 minutes
- Cook Time: 60 minutes
- Total Time: 65 minutes
- Serving: 4

<u>Ingredients</u>

- ¼ lb dried chickpeas (soaked in water for one night)

- 1½ tablespoon tahini
- 1 tablespoon lemon juice
- 2 tablespoons extra virgin olive oil, divided
- ¼ teaspoon cumin
- ½ teaspoon salt
- 1 tablespoon water
- 1 teaspoon baking soda (optional)
- 1 teaspoon paprika powder (optional)
- ½ teaspoon garlic powder (optional)

<u>Instructions</u>

1. First, people with fructose intolerance need to soak the chickpeas overnight in water and optionally add baking soda to the water.
2. Cook your chickpeas in a large pot with water, over medium heat for about one hour. Check if chickpeas cooked well by crushing one of them with a fork in your hand.
3. When chickpeas cooked, drain them and put them in a blender.
4. Add 1 tablespoon of extra virgin olive oil, lemon juice, tahini, cumin powder, salt, and garlic powder (optional) to the blender. Blend until your hummus gets a soft, creamy texture equally.
5. Sprinkle with one tablespoon extra virgin olive oil or paprika powder (optional).
6. Serve immediately or fridge it.

<u>Cooking Tips:</u>

- You can serve hummus, hot or cold.

<u>Fructose Intolerance-related Tips:</u>

- Do not use paprika and garlic powders in hummus if you are experiencing a severe flare-up.
- Eat hummus in moderation. It is better to avoid making Hummus during flares, or make and eat a little bit of it.

Nutrition Facts
Servings: 4

Amount per serving	
Calories	**198**
	% Daily Value*
Total Fat 11.8g	15%
Saturated Fat 1.6g	8%
Cholesterol 0mg	0%
Sodium 305mg	13%
Total Carbohydrate 18.5g	7%
Dietary Fiber 5.5g	20%
Total Sugars 3.1g	
Protein 6.5g	
Vitamin D 0mcg	0%
Calcium 56mg	4%
Iron 2mg	13%
Potassium 279mg	6%

Tofu

Tofu is a fantastic snack option for people with fructose intolerance. It is based on soy milk and is rich in calcium and Iron, needed for most people with fructose intolerance. Here is a sample recipe of a snack with Tofu:

Avocado Tofu Toast

Enjoy a healthy and rich daily snack!

- Prep Time: 10 minutes
- Cook Time: 35 minutes
- Total Time: 45 minutes
- Serving: 4

Ingredients

- 1½ cup firm tofu, pressed and drained

- 1 avocado, cubed
- 1 tablespoon extra virgin olive oil
- ½ teaspoon garlic powder (optional)
- Salt and pepper, to taste

<u>Instructions</u>

1. Preheat your oven to 400 °F.
2. Choose a baking sheet, cover it with parchment paper or spray extra virgin olive oil. Cut tofu-like cubes of 1.5 inches and spray extra virgin olive oil on it.
3. Let it bake for 15 minutes until golden brown and crispy. Flip tofu and cook for another 10 minutes. Remove from the oven. Let it rest for 10 minutes.
4. Cube avocado on a plate and add garlic powder (optional), salt, and pepper.
5. Mix the tofu with avocado in a bowl. Enjoy!

<u>Cooking Tips:</u>

- You may want to add one tablespoon of lemon juice to create another great taste.

<u>Fructose Intolerance-related Tips:</u>

- Do not use pepper and garlic powder in this toast if you are experiencing a flare-up.

Nutrition Facts	
Servings: 4	
Amount per serving	
Calories	**199**
	% Daily Value*
Total Fat 17.2g	22%
Saturated Fat 3.4g	17%
Cholesterol 0mg	0%
Sodium 14mg	1%
Total Carbohydrate 5.9g	2%
Dietary Fiber 4.2g	15%
Total Sugars 0.8g	
Protein 8.7g	
Vitamin D 0mcg	0%
Calcium 196mg	15%
Iron 2mg	10%
Potassium 384mg	8%

ALMOND BUTTER SANDWICH

Almond butter is a fantastic source of fiber and magnesium for people with fructose intolerance. It is recommended to use smooth almond butter.

- Prep Time: 5 minutes
- Total Time: 5 minutes
- Serving: 1

Ingredients

- 2 slices of gluten-free bread
- 1 tablespoon organic smooth almond butter

Instructions

1. Spread one piece of bread with almond butter.
2. Toast and enjoy!

Cooking Tips:

- You can combine the almond butter sandwich with almond milk or lactose-free cow milk perfectly.

Fructose Intolerance-related Tips:

- Remember to use smooth almond butter.

Nutrition Facts	
Servings: 1	
Amount per serving	
Calories	**313**
	% Daily Value*
Total Fat 17.7g	23%
Saturated Fat 1.9g	9%
Cholesterol 0mg	0%
Sodium 341mg	15%
Total Carbohydrate 32.3g	12%
Dietary Fiber 5.2g	19%
Total Sugars 4.2g	
Protein 8.8g	
Vitamin D 0mcg	0%
Calcium 156mg	12%
Iron 3mg	16%
Potassium 280mg	6%

GLUTEN-FREE MUFFINS

You may eat different types of muffins, but you have to make sure about the ingredients. The muffin should not be made with fruits you cannot tolerate. Moreover, try not to eat muffins that are made with whole wheat flour. If you are gluten-intolerant or suffering from fructose intolerance, you can make your muffins at home:

- Prep Time: 15 minutes
- Cook Time: 45 minutes
- Total Time: 60 minutes
- Serving: 5-10 (10 Muffins)

<u>Ingredients</u>

- 2 tablespoons extra virgin olive oil or avocado oil
- 2½ cups almond flour, blanched
- 3 large organic free-range eggs
- ¼ cup organic brown sugar
- 2 teaspoons vanilla extract
- ¼ cup banana, mashed
- 1 teaspoon lemon juice

- ¾ teaspoon baking soda
- ¼ teaspoon cinnamon powder
- ½ teaspoon salt

<u>Instructions</u>

1. Preheat your oven to 375 °F.
2. In a large bowl, mix almond flour, cinnamon, baking soda, and salt. Whisk well.
3. In another bowl, add extra virgin olive oil, vanilla extract, eggs, banana, brown sugar, and lemon juice. Whisk well.
4. Mix the two bowls and stir well with a wooden spoon until flour mixed well with other ingredients.
5. Prepare ten muffin cups. Pour them to the top and then bake for 15 minutes.
6. To avoid browning quickly, loosely cover muffins with an aluminum foil. Cook for another 15 minutes.
7. Put a toothpick in a muffin to check if it cooks well or not. If cooked well, the toothpick should not stick to the muffin.
8. Remove from the oven. Let the muffins cool for 15 more minutes. Enjoy!

<u>Cooking Tips:</u>

- You need to use finely grounded flour.

Nutrition Facts	
Servings: 10	
Amount per serving	
Calories	**366**
	% Daily Value*
Total Fat 30.7g	39%
Saturated Fat 2.9g	14%
Cholesterol 65mg	22%
Sodium 242mg	11%
Total Carbohydrate 16.1g	6%
Dietary Fiber 5.1g	18%
Total Sugars 7.8g	
Protein 12.8g	
Vitamin D 0mcg	0%
Calcium 132mg	10%
Iron 2mg	11%
Potassium 31mg	1%

CHEESE STICKS

Cheese sticks are excellent sources of calcium. You may consume lactose-free cheese sticks as snacks. Remember to choose low fat or fat-free options. If you are lactose-intolerant, you may use lactose-free Swiss, Havarti, or aged cheddar. One cheddar cheese sticks have the following nutrition fact:

Nutrition Facts	
Servings: 1	
Amount per serving	
Calories	**110**
	% Daily Value*
Total Fat 9g	12%
Saturated Fat 5g	25%
Cholesterol 30mg	10%
Sodium 180mg	8%
Total Carbohydrate 0g	0%
Dietary Fiber 0g	0%
Total Sugars 0g	
Protein 7g	
Vitamin D 0mcg	0%
Calcium 200mg	15%
Iron 0mg	0%
Potassium 0mg	0%

AVOCADO TUNA TOAST

A very fast sandwich you can prepare at home.

- Prep Time: 10 minutes

- Cook Time: 0 minutes
- Total Time: 10 minutes
- Serving: 4

Ingredients

- 2 avocados
- 2 tablespoons organic low-fat mayonnaise
- 1 teaspoon cumin powder
- 1 can of tuna in olive oil or water
- 4 white gluten-free toasts
- Salt to taste
- 1 teaspoon Dijon mustard (optional)
- Pepper to taste (optional)

Instructions

1. Choose a small bowl. Mix tuna with smashed avocado with mayo, cumin powder, mustard (optional), salt, and pepper (optional).
2. Place tuna mix on two toast slices. Cover with other slices.
3. Toast and enjoy!

Cooking Tips:

- You can make this sandwich without mayonnaise sauce, as well.

Fructose Intolerance-related Tips:

- Do not use black pepper or cumin powder if you are experiencing a flare-up.

Nutrition Facts	
Servings: 4	
Amount per serving	
Calories	**386**
	% Daily Value*
Total Fat 26.7g	34%
Saturated Fat 5.2g	26%
Cholesterol 17mg	6%
Sodium 268mg	12%
Total Carbohydrate 23.3g	8%
Dietary Fiber 7.7g	27%
Total Sugars 3g	
Protein 15.8g	
Vitamin D 0mcg	0%
Calcium 45mg	3%
Iron 2mg	11%
Potassium 689mg	15%

RICE CRACKERS

Most rice crackers in the market are gluten-free and good snacks for people with fructose intolerance. White rice is an excellent carbohydrate for people with fructose intolerance.

GLUTEN-FREE RICE CRACKER

A great example of making a rice cracker as a snack.

- Prep Time: 10 minutes
- Cook Time: 15 minutes
- Total Time: 25 minutes
- Serving: 6

Ingredients

- 1 cup white rice flour
- 2 tablespoons extra virgin olive oil
- ⅓ cup of water
- ½ tablespoon salt
- 1 teaspoon brown sugar (optional)

Instructions

1. Preheat oven to 350 °F.

2. In a large bowl, mix white rice flour with oil, salt, brown sugar, and water to create a smooth dough.
3. Roll out the dough on a floured surface and make round, thin rice cookies.
4. Make holes throughout rice cookies by using a fork. Spray them with extra virgin olive oil.
5. Bake crackers for about 15 minutes until slightly golden. Enjoy!

<u>Cooking Tips:</u>

- You can make this cracker in a large pan, as well. Just bake them with extra virgin olive oil over low heat until golden both sides.

<u>Fructose Intolerance-related Tips:</u>

- Make sure you are using white rice flour and no other types of rice flours such as brown rice flours.

Nutrition Facts

Servings: 6

Amount per serving

Calories	**190**

	% Daily Value*
Total Fat 5.2g	7%
Saturated Fat 0.7g	3%
Cholesterol 0mg	0%
Sodium 582mg	25%
Total Carbohydrate 32g	12%
Dietary Fiber 1g	4%
Total Sugars 0g	
Protein 2g	
Vitamin D 0mcg	0%
Calcium 1mg	0%
Iron 0mg	0%
Potassium 0mg	0%

GINSENG BISCUITS

Ginseng is rich in potassium and vitamin B6 with excellent anti-inflammatory properties. Hence, ginseng-based snacks are great snack options for people with fructose intolerance.

GLUTEN-FREE GINSENG BISCUITS

Enjoy making a gluten-free, dairy-free ginseng biscuit in your home, perfectly matched to fructose intolerance conditions.

- Prep Time: 15 minutes
- Cook Time: 20 minutes
- Total Time: 35 minutes
- Serving: 4-6

<u>Ingredients</u>

- ¾ cup shortening or half a cup + 1 tablespoon extra virgin olive oil
- 2 cups gluten-free flour or grated almond flour
- 2 tablespoons brown sugar
- 1 organic, free-range egg
- 2 teaspoons baking soda
- ¼ cup molasses
- 1½ teaspoons freshly grated ginseng
- 1 teaspoon cinnamon powder
- ½ teaspoon salt

<u>Instructions</u>

1. In a large bowl, mix oil (or shortening), sugar, molasses, and egg.
2. In another large bowl, mix flour, ginseng, baking soda, cinnamon, and salt.
3. Slowly combine ingredients of both bowls until making a soft dough.
4. Let the dough rest for 45 minutes.
5. Preheat oven to 375°F.

6. Roll the dough and make 2-inch (5cm) balls. Pour maple syrup on dough balls.
7. Use cookie sheets with parchment paper. Put balls on cooking sheets and bake for 12-15 minutes until seeing cracks and until having a light brown color.
8. Remove from the oven and cool biscuits for five minutes. Enjoy!

<u>Cooking Tips:</u>

- Shortening gives you a better ginseng biscuit texture. However, people with fructose intolerance may not tolerate it well. Alternatively, use olive oil.
- You can substitute ¼ cup of molasses with ¼ cup brown sugar.

<u>Fructose Intolerance-related Tips:</u>

- Do not use molasses if you cannot tolerate it. Instead, use brown sugar.

Nutrition Facts

Servings: 6

Amount per serving

Calories	367
	% Daily Value*
Total Fat 4.5g	6%
Saturated Fat 1.1g	5%
Cholesterol 27mg	9%
Sodium 660mg	29%
Total Carbohydrate 77.2g	28%
Dietary Fiber 8.5g	30%
Total Sugars 15.3g	
Protein 5.6g	
Vitamin D 3mcg	13%
Calcium 34mg	3%
Iron 1mg	6%
Potassium 236mg	5%

ZUCCHINI CHIPS

Zucchini chips are a healthy, low-calorie snack for people with fructose intolerance with lots of crunchiness as well as vitamin C and B6!

- Prep Time: 20 minutes
- Cook Time: 90 minutes
- Total Time: 110 minutes
- Serving: 2-4

Ingredients

- 2 zucchinis, sliced thin
- 1 tablespoon extra virgin olive oil
- Salt, to taste
- ¼ teaspoon cumin powder (optional)
- ½ teaspoon garlic powder (optional)

Instructions

1- Slice zucchinis lengthwise and thin by a slicer.
2- Take out the moisture from zucchinis using clean paper towels. Hold and press down paper towels on zucchinis.
3- Preheat the over to 250 °F.
4- Spray olive oil on parchment papers and then, place zucchinis on them.
5- Spray or pour olive oil on top of zucchinis as well. Sprinkle salt, cumin powder (optional) and garlic powder (optional).
6- Bake zucchinis for about 80-90 minutes until golden.
7- Remove from the oven. Dry zucchinis with a paper towel. Enjoy!

Cooking Tips:

- You can also fry zucchinis in a large pan by extra virgin olive oil over low heat or microwave it. For more crispiness, you may need to broil fried zucchinis.

<u>Fructose Intolerance-related Tips:</u>

- Do not use garlic powder if you cannot tolerate it or if you have a flare-up.

Nutrition Facts	
Servings: 2	
Amount per serving	
Calories	**95**
	% Daily Value*
Total Fat 7.4g	10%
Saturated Fat 1.1g	5%
Cholesterol 0mg	0%
Sodium 20mg	1%
Total Carbohydrate 7.2g	3%
Dietary Fiber 2.3g	8%
Total Sugars 3.6g	
Protein 2.5g	
Vitamin D 0mcg	0%
Calcium 32mg	2%
Iron 1mg	5%
Potassium 526mg	11%

HEALTHY POTATO CHIPS

Crunchy and healthy potato chips can be a tasty snack for people with fructose intolerance as they can be made with no oil, and as the snack is fat-free.

- Prep Time: 10 minutes
- Cook Time: 10 minutes
- Total Time: 20 minutes
- Serving: 2

<u>Ingredients</u>

- 2 medium potatoes, skin removed
- ½ teaspoon garlic powder (optional)

- ½ teaspoon onion powder (optional)
- Salt, to taste

Instructions

1. Wash potatoes and then, peel-off the skins.
2. Slice potatoes into chips using a very thin slicer.
3. Add salt, garlic powder (optional), and onion powder (optional).
4. Spread all chips on a parchment paper sheet.
5. Put in the microwave until golden brown. Enjoy!

Cooking Tips:

- Potato chips perfectly match with any avocado snack.

Fructose Intolerance-related Tips:

- Do not use garlic or onion powder when you are experiencing a flare-up. Make chips with salt only.

Nutrition Facts

Servings: 2

Amount per serving

Calories	151
	% Daily Value*
Total Fat 0.2g	0%
Saturated Fat 0.1g	0%
Cholesterol 0mg	0%
Sodium 13mg	1%
Total Carbohydrate 34.5g	13%
Dietary Fiber 5.2g	19%
Total Sugars 2.8g	
Protein 3.8g	
Vitamin D 0mcg	0%
Calcium 22mg	2%
Iron 1mg	6%
Potassium 880mg	19%

DRINKS

RECOMMENDED HOT BEVERAGES

Recommended hot beverages for people with fructose intolerance are:

- <u>Decaffeinated coffee:</u> use decaffeinated coffee instead of caffeinated coffee if you are experiencing a flare-up. It is recommended not to take caffeinated drinks at all if you can.

- <u>Decaffeinated black tea:</u> if you would like to have earl gray, English breakfast, or any types of black tea, it is better to drink decaffeinated kinds, especially if you are experiencing a flare-up. If you are in remission, take caffeinated black tea in moderation. As cinnamon has anti-inflammatory properties, it is a great idea to pour a little bit of cinnamon powder in your black tea.

- <u>Peppermint Tea:</u> this herbal tea is an excellent choice for people with fructose intolerance as it has properties that can soothe your digestive tract. Studies show that peppermint oil can help spasms and cramping in patients with gastrointestinal issues.

- <u>Green Tea:</u> is another excellent choice for people with fructose intolerance. It includes polyphenol antioxidants such as epigallocatechin gallate (EGCG), a type of catechin that protects cells from damages and can reduce inflammation or irritation that helps chronic conditions. It can also help inhibit bacterial growth, which lowers the risks of getting infections. Moreover, green tea contains less caffeine than regular coffee. However, it could give you a similar mood.

- <u>Ziziphora/Oregano/Thyme Tea:</u> This herbal tea is recommended for people with fructose intolerance. Ziziphora is the name of a mountain plant from the Lamiaceae group, similar to Thyme. It has flavonoids with anti-inflammatory properties. Oregano contains great antioxidants such as Carvacrol and Thymol that can reduce the risk of virus activities. Studies have shown excellent anti-inflammatory properties of oregano. Thyme tea is also great for people with fructose intolerance. It has antioxidants and antimicrobial properties with valuable sources of Iron. Thyme can also be used in foods as a great seasoning. You can pour one tablespoon of Ziziphora or Oregano or Thyme in a cup of boiling water and enjoy drinking this fantastic tea after 8-10 minutes.

- <u>Turmeric and Ginseng Tea:</u> both turmeric and ginseng are fantastic for people living with fructose intolerance. Turmeric and Ginseng have been used widely in ancient medicine. They use turmeric and ginseng as medicines and for better digestion. Turmeric is high in antioxidants that can protect your cells from damaging and reduces the risks of getting infections. Curcumin in turmeric is a great anti-inflammatory ingredient. Ginseng also has strong properties that can help reduce inflammation in the GI tract.

  - For making a great tea, add ½ teaspoon of ground turmeric and ½ teaspoon of freshly grated ginseng in 2 cups of boiling water and enjoy your drink after 12-15 minutes. You can add 1-teaspoon brown sugar to your tea if you can tolerate it.

One of the delicious hot beverages you can make with Turmeric and Ginseng is called Golden-like Milk:

  - Golden-like Milk: mix ½ cup of unsweetened almond milk or lactose-free cow milk, one teaspoon turmeric, ½ teaspoon of freshly grated ginseng, ½ teaspoon of cinnamon powder, and one teaspoon of maple syrup (optional: if you can tolerate) in a small pot and boil. After boiling, simmer for 5 minutes until flavors over low heat.

- <u>Mint Tea:</u> you can benefit from mint properties by making this great tea. Mint has menthol, which helps reduce inflammation in the gut. Boil 10-15 mint leaves with one tablespoon of lemon juice and 2 cups of water in a small pot. Remove from heat, wait for three more minutes and add one tablespoon maple syrup (optional: if you can tolerate) for sweetness if you want.

- <u>Slippery Elm Tea:</u> recent studies showed that slippery elm bark could soothe the stomach and intestinal linings and reducing irritations and might be an excellent drink for people with fructose intolerance. Pour one tablespoon of slippery elm in a cup of boiling water and enjoy drinking after 10 minutes.

- <u>Calendula Tea:</u> this tea is known for helping people with peptic ulcers, reflux, and IBD. It can soothe gut inflammation and/or irritation as it has anti-inflammatory and wound-healing properties. Pour 1 tablespoon of dried calendula in a cup of boiling water and enjoy drinking after 10-12 minutes.

- <u>Milk:</u> Generally speaking, some people with fructose intolerance cannot tolerate lactose in cow milk.
  - Some researchers recommend not to use regular cow milk or any nut/wild rice milk at all when you are in a flare-up as milk is a hard-to-digest drink.

o If you are in remission, it is recommended to consume low-fat lactose-free cow milk, unsweetened almond milk, or rice milk. You can also use soy milk during remissions, but make sure you are using a Non-GMO type. Always check your intolerance level.

RECOMMENDED COLD BEVERAGES

Recommended cold beverages for people with fructose intolerance are as below:

- <u>Water:</u> The best drink for people with fructose intolerance is water. Try drinking at least 8-10 glasses of water each day, especially if you are experiencing a flare-up, which helps relieve your diarrhea.
  - o Some patients experienced better feelings of consuming alkaline water with 9.5 pH. Alkaline water is water with a pH of more than 7 (normal). As it has a higher pH than regular water, some claim that it can balance body pH level. Most soda drinks in the market have acidic properties (pH smaller than 7). Ionized alkaline water can increase hydration as ionization may reduce the size of molecular clusters of water. Some experts also claimed that as active oxygen in water is a free radical, it might damage healthy tissues. Alkaline water may neutralize active oxygen and avoid those damaging healthy tissues.
- <u>Do not drink</u> sweet soda, carbonated beverages, and caffeinated beverages if you have fructose

intolerance. These drinks may cause you diarrhea and bloating, and can trigger your symptoms.

- <u>Gatorade/Powerade:</u> is a fantastic electrolyte drink for people with fructose intolerance. It can help to relieve diarrhea, and it contains useful minerals such as sodium, potassium, and vitamins such as B3, B6, and B12.
    - o When you are in flare-up periods, try your electrolyte recipe: First glass: mix one cup of water with ½ teaspoon of sugar and a pinch of salt. Second glass: mix one cup of boiled water with ¼ teaspoon of baking soda. When in hydration, drink half of the first glass and then half of the second glass. Drink more from glasses, respectively, if you are still thirsty.
- <u>Fruit Juices:</u> Fruit juices are excellent sources of vitamins for people with fructose intolerance. Juicing from tolerable fruits is essential for people with fructose intolerance. Hence, they can boost their nutrient intake by juicing. However, people with fructose intolerance need to consume specific fruits with specific instructions:
    - o It is recommended not to add sugar or any artificial sweeteners to juices. If you can tolerate brown sugar, you can add it to your juice.
    - o Make sure peeling off fruit skins when you are juicing them. Typically fruit skins are hard to digest.
    - o It is recommended to consume only tolerable fruits/ fruit juices.
    - o The best fruit juice that can be consumed in moderation by people with fructose

intolerance are Aloe Vera, Papaya, Carrot, Cantaloupe, Pineapples, Blackberries, Peach, Strawberries, Pumpkin, and Nectarine.

- o You may want to try other fruit juices (skin removed) when you are in remission. You may also juice vegetables such as celery and spinach during your remission period. Always start consuming less and check your tolerance level.
- o Many experts recommend eating berries such as blueberries and strawberries.
- o Most people with fructose intolerance cannot tolerate tomato juice. Try not to consume it, especially if you are in a flare.

It is better to purchase organic fruits and always correctly wash fruits first, even if you know that you want to remove their skins.

CHAPTER 4. BI-WEEKLY COOKING PLAN

This chapter provides you with examples of biweekly meal plans. It can give you an idea of how to create your biweekly plans. Here are some of the essential tips you need to remember when you want to make your meal plan:

- Try varieties of non-triggering foods, but always eat and drink healthy foods.
- If you are lactose-intolerant, try alternative products explained in this book.
- If you are gluten-intolerant, try alternative products explained in this book.
- It is recommended to fully avoid consuming lactose and gluten.
- Remember: when you are in a flare, you have to put more anti-inflammatory non-triggering soups, juices, and broth in your meal plan. Keep yourself hydrated.
- Put more foods with anti-inflammatory herbs and spices such as turmeric in your flare-up meal plan as well.
- Drink safe herbal teas such as peppermint and green tea.
- If you are sensitive to seafood, you can substitute seafood with other foods with healthy fat and protein sources. This book gives you different non-seafood cooking recipes.
- When you are in remission (when it seems that your symptoms are gone!), it does not mean that you can eat everything. There are still some triggering foods for you to avoid as they can wake up flares. Always make your meal plan based on your health conditions

and non-triggering foods that can be well-tolerated by you.

- Remember that it is recommended to eat six portions a day instead of three portions. Hence, you can have breakfast, snack (between breakfast and lunch), lunch, snack (between lunch and dinner), dinner, and snack (between dinner and your sleep time). You can use appetizers, snacks, desserts, and snack recipes in this book for the snack portions. Alternatively, you can have soups or salads as before-lunch or before-dinner snacks.
- If you have issues in making an effective meal plan for yourself, you can always ask support from a nutritionist or a dietitian.

Here are two examples of your "Biweekly Meal Plan":

Week-1:	Week-2:
Monday	Monday
Breakfast: Avocado Egg Breakfast Toast **Snack-1:** Zucchini Chips **Lunch:** Chicken Kebab (From Last Night) **Snack-2:** Banana Milkshake **Dinner:** Grilled Salmon and/or Carrot Potato Soup **Snack-3:** Diced Fruits **Drinks:** Coffee, Peppermint Tea	**Breakfast:** Egg Tacos with Avocado **Snack-1:** Gluten-Free Rice Crackers **Lunch:** Chicken Stroganoff (From Last Night) **Snack-2:** Almond Butter Toast **Dinner:** Lemon Steamed Halibut with White Rice **Snack-3:** Banana Ginseng Sundae **Drinks:** Earl Gray Tea, Green Tea
Tuesday	Tuesday
Breakfast: Almond Butter Banana Sandwich **Snack-1:** Gluten-Free Ginseng Biscuit **Lunch:** Grilled Salmon and/or Carrot Potato Soup **Snack-2:** Avocado Smoothie **Dinner:** Potato Cutlet with Stracciatella Soup **Snack-3:** Rice cracker **Drinks:** Decaffeinated Black Tea, Green Tea	**Breakfast:** Fruit Salad with Almond Milk **Snack-1:** Avocado Dip **Lunch:** Lemon Steamed Halibut with White Rice **Snack-2:** Banana Cinnamon Smoothie **Dinner:** Classic Tuna Pasta Salad or Pumpkin Soup **Snack-3:** Pomegranate Angelica Smoothie **Drinks:** Decaffeinated Coffee, Peppermint Tea
Wednesday	Wednesday
Breakfast: Strawberry Cinnamon Oatmeal **Snack-1:** Tofu Toast **Lunch:** Potato Cutlet with Stracciatella Soup **Snack-2:** Cantaloupe Smoothie **Dinner:** Pineapple Pork **Snack-3:** Poached Fruit Compote **Drinks:** Decaffeinated Coffee, Peppermint Tea	**Breakfast:** Pineapple Ginseng Oatmeal **Snack-1:** Guacamole-Like Snack **Lunch:** Classic Tuna Pasta Salad or Pumpkin Soup **Snack-2:** Banana Milkshake **Dinner:** Olivier/Potato Salad **Snack-3:** Cantaloupe Mix Smoothie **Drinks:** Coffee, Oregano Tea
Thursday	Thursday
Breakfast: Gluten-Free Fluffy Pancakes **Snack-1:** Lactose Free Cheese Sticks **Lunch:** Pineapple Pork **Snack-2:** Blueberry Pineapple Banana Smoothie **Dinner:** Thunfisch Pizza and **Snack-3:** Strawberry Pie **Drinks:** Black Tea with Cinnamon, Ginseng Mint Tea	**Breakfast:** Baked Pineapple **Snack-1:** Avocado Cheese Bagel **Lunch:** Olivier/Potato Salad **Snack-2:** Baba Ghanoush **Dinner:** Grilled Beef Kebab with White Rice **Snack-3:** Carrot Juice with Pineapple Ice Cream **Drinks:** Decaffeinated Earl Grey Tea, Ginseng Mint Tea
Friday	Friday
Breakfast: Two Poached Eggs with Toasts **Snack-1:** Almond Butter Sandwich **Lunch:** Thunfisch Pizza and **Snack-2:** Banana Cinnamon Smoothie	**Breakfast:** Almond Butter Banana Toast **Snack-1:** Rice cracker **Lunch:** Grilled Beef Kebab with White Rice

Dinner: Chicken Zucchini Stew with Chicken Broth **Snack-3:** Diced Fruits such as Papaya **Drinks:** Decaffeinated Coffee, Ziziphora Tea	**Snack-2:** Carrot Avocado Salad **Dinner:** Chicken Pineapple Pizza **Snack-3:** Warm Pineapple Crumble **Drinks:** Decaffeinated Coffee, Green Tea
Saturday	Saturday
Breakfast: Avocado Cheese Bagel **Snack-1:** Poached Fruits with Lactose-Free Plain Yogurt **Lunch:** Chicken Zucchini Stew with Chicken Broth **Snack-2:** Butter Lettuce Salad **Dinner:** Hungarian Goulash with Bone Broth **Snack-3:** Lemon Sorbet or a Fruit Juice **Drinks:** Coffee, Turmeric Ginseng Tea	**Breakfast:** Egg Salmon Avocado **Snack-1:** Tofu Toast **Lunch:** Chicken Pineapple Pizza **Snack-2:** Avocado Smoothie **Dinner:** Chicken & Shrimp Teriyaki with Rice Noodles **Snack-3:** Rice Pudding **Drinks:** Coffee, Turmeric Ginseng Tea
Sunday	Sunday
Breakfast: Smoothie Bowl with Almond Milk **Snack-1:** Gluten-Free Rice Crackers **Lunch:** Hungarian Goulash with Bone Broth **Snack-2:** Hummus **Dinner:** Chicken Stroganoff **Snack-3:** Avocado Blueberry Popsicle **Drinks:** Decaffeinated Coffee, Slippery Elm Tea	**Breakfast:** Zucchini Bread Oatmeal **Snack-1:** Gluten-Free Ginseng Biscuit **Lunch:** Chicken & Shrimp Teriyaki with Rice Noodles **Snack-2:** Pineapple Papaya Salad **Dinner:** Ginseng Sticky Pork **Snack-3:** Pineapple Cake Sundae **Drinks:** Decaffeinated Black Tea, Calendula Tea

Week-1:	Week-2:
Monday	**Monday**
Breakfast: Avocado + 2 Poached Eggs **Snack-1:** Zucchini Salad **Lunch:** Chicken Kebab with White Rice (From Last Night) **Snack-2:** Carrot Juice **Dinner:** Boiled Salmon / Carrot Potato Soup **Snack-3:** Diced Non-Triggering Fruits **Drinks:** Decaffeinated Coffee, Peppermint Tea	**Breakfast:** Two Poached Eggs with Avocado **Snack-1:** Avocado Dip **Lunch:** Chicken Noodle Soup (From Last Night) **Snack-2:** Banana smoothie **Dinner:** Lemon Steamed Halibut with White Rice **Snack-3:** Ginseng Fruit Sherbet (Sweetened by brown sugar) **Drinks:** Decaffeinated Black Tea, Green Tea
Tuesday	**Tuesday**
Breakfast: Smooth Almond Butter Banana Sandwich **Snack-1:** Gluten-Free Ginseng Biscuit or Rice Crackers **Lunch:** Boiled Salmon / Carrot Potato Soup **Snack-2:** Cantaloupe Juice **Dinner:** Turkey Pot Pie Soup **Snack-3:** Rice crackers **Drinks:** Decaffeinated Black Tea, Green Tea	**Breakfast:** Fruit Salad **Snack-1:** Oatmeal (if tolerable) or Firm Tofu **Lunch:** Lemon Steamed Halibut with White Rice **Snack-2:** Carrot Juice **Dinner:** Classic Tuna Pasta Salad + One Bone Broth Cup **Snack-3:** Pomegranate Angelica Drink **Drinks:** Decaffeinated Coffee, Peppermint Tea
Wednesday	**Wednesday**
Breakfast: Oatmeal (if tolerable) or Safe Fruit Bowl **Snack-1:** Firm Tofu Toast **Lunch:** Turkey Pot Pie Soup **Snack-2:** Cantaloupe Juice **Dinner:** Bone Broth + Carrot Avocado Salad **Snack-3:** Poached Fruit Compote **Drinks:** Green Tea, Peppermint Tea	**Breakfast:** Oatmeal (if tolerable) or a Safe Fruit Bowl **Snack-1:** Guacamole-Like Snack **Lunch:** Classic Tuna Pasta Salad + One Bone Broth Cup **Snack-2:** Diced Banana **Dinner:** Potato Salad + Pumpkin Soup **Snack-3:** Cantaloupe Juice **Drinks:** Green Tea, Peppermint Tea
Thursday	**Thursday**
Breakfast: Two Poached Eggs with Toasts **Snack-1:** Diced Fruits **Lunch:** Bone Broth + Carrot Avocado Salad **Snack-2:** Avocado Smoothie (Lactose-Free) **Dinner:** Stracciatella Soup **Snack-3:** Cantaloupe Juice **Drinks:** Decaffeinated Black Tea, Ginseng Mint Tea	**Breakfast:** Baked Pineapple **Snack-1:** Smooth Almond Butter Sandwich **Lunch:** Potato Salad + Pumpkin Soup **Snack-2:** Poached Egg Avocado White Pita **Dinner:** Turkey Zucchini Noodles **Snack-3:** Carrot Juice **Drinks:** Decaffeinated Earl Grey Tea, Ginseng Mint Tea
Friday	**Friday**
Breakfast: Avocado + Gluten-Free Bagel	**Breakfast:** Almond Butter Banana Toast

Snack-1: Almond Butter Sandwich **Lunch:** Stracciatella Soup **Snack-2:** Rice crackers **Dinner:** Chicken Zucchini Stew with Chicken Broth **Snack-3:** Diced Fruits such as Papaya **Drinks:** Decaffeinated Coffee, Peppermint Tea	**Snack-1:** rice crackers **Lunch:** Turkey Zucchini Noodles **Snack-2:** Carrot Avocado Salad **Dinner:** Pumpkin Soup **Snack-3:** Lemon Sorbet **Drinks:** Peppermint Tea, Green Tea
Saturday	Saturday
Breakfast: Smooth Almond Butter Banana Sandwich **Snack-1:** Poached Fruits (Unsweetened or with brown sugar) **Lunch:** Chicken Zucchini Stew with Chicken Broth **Snack-2:** Ginseng Cool Drink **Dinner:** Bone Broth and Mashed Potato with No Milk **Snack-3:** Lemon Sorbet **Drinks:** Turmeric Ginseng Tea, Turmeric Ginseng Tea	**Breakfast:** 2 Poached Eggs with Avocado **Snack-1:** Firm Tofu Toast **Lunch:** Pumpkin Soup **Snack-2:** Papaya Dices **Dinner:** Lemon Shrimp with White Rice **Snack-3:** Rice Pudding (Unsweetened or by brown sugar) **Drinks:** Decaffeinated Coffee, Turmeric Ginseng Tea
Sunday	Sunday
Breakfast: Smoothie Bowl with Almond Milk **Snack-1:** Gluten-Free Rice Crackers **Lunch:** Bone Broth and Mashed Potato with No Milk **Snack-2:** Guacamole Like Snack **Dinner:** Chicken Noodle Soup **Snack-3:** Popsicle from a Non-triggering Fruit **Drinks:** Decaffeinated Coffee, Green Tea	**Breakfast:** Zucchini Bread Oatmeal **Snack-1:** Gluten-Free Ginseng Biscuit **Lunch:** Lemon Shrimp with White Rice **Snack-2:** Pineapple Papaya Salad **Dinner:** Zucchini Salad **Snack-3:** Popsicle from a Non-triggering Fruit **Drinks:** Decaffeinated Black Tea, Peppermint Tea

BIWEEKLY COOKING PLAN – BLANK

This section gives you two free blank meal plan tables that can be filled by you when you want to create your own biweekly plans.

<table>
<tr><th colspan="2">Biweekly Meal Plan - 1</th></tr>
<tr><td>Week-1:</td><td>Week-2:</td></tr>
<tr><td>Monday</td><td>Monday</td></tr>
<tr><td>Breakfast:
Snack-1:
Lunch:
Snack-2:
Dinner:
Snack-3:
Drinks:</td><td>Breakfast:
Snack-1:
Lunch:
Snack-2:
Dinner:
Snack-3:
Drinks:</td></tr>
<tr><td>Tuesday</td><td>Tuesday</td></tr>
<tr><td>Breakfast:
Snack-1:
Lunch:
Snack-2:
Dinner:
Snack-3:
Drinks:</td><td>Breakfast:
Snack-1:
Lunch:
Snack-2:
Dinner:
Snack-3:
Drinks:</td></tr>
<tr><td>Wednesday</td><td>Wednesday</td></tr>
<tr><td>Breakfast:
Snack-1:
Lunch:
Snack-2:
Dinner:
Snack-3:
Drinks:</td><td>Breakfast:
Snack-1:
Lunch:
Snack-2:
Dinner:
Snack-3:
Drinks:</td></tr>
<tr><td>Thursday</td><td>Thursday</td></tr>
<tr><td>Breakfast:
Snack-1:
Lunch:
Snack-2:
Dinner:
Snack-3:
Drinks:</td><td>Breakfast:
Snack-1:
Lunch:
Snack-2:
Dinner:
Snack-3:
Drinks:</td></tr>
<tr><td>Friday</td><td>Friday</td></tr>
<tr><td>Breakfast:
Snack-1:
Lunch:
Snack-2:
Dinner:
Snack-3:
Drinks:</td><td>Breakfast:
Snack-1:
Lunch:
Snack-2:
Dinner:
Snack-3:
Drinks:</td></tr>
<tr><td>Saturday</td><td>Saturday</td></tr>
<tr><td>Breakfast:
Snack-1:
Lunch:
Snack-2:
Dinner:
Snack-3:
Drinks:</td><td>Breakfast:
Snack-1:
Lunch:
Snack-2:
Dinner:
Snack-3:
Drinks:</td></tr>
<tr><td>Sunday</td><td>Sunday</td></tr>
<tr><td>Breakfast:
Snack-1:
Lunch:
Snack-2:
Dinner:
Snack-3:
Drinks:</td><td>Breakfast:
Snack-1:
Lunch:
Snack-2:
Dinner:
Snack-3:
Drinks:</td></tr>
</table>

Biweekly Meal Plan - 2	
Week-1:	**Week-2:**
Monday	Monday
Breakfast: **Snack-1:** **Lunch:** **Snack-2:** **Dinner:** **Snack-3:** **Drinks:**	**Breakfast:** **Snack-1:** **Lunch:** **Snack-2:** **Dinner:** **Snack-3:** **Drinks:**
Tuesday	Tuesday
Breakfast: **Snack-1:** **Lunch:** **Snack-2:** **Dinner:** **Snack-3:** **Drinks:**	**Breakfast:** **Snack-1:** **Lunch:** **Snack-2:** **Dinner:** **Snack-3:** **Drinks:**
Wednesday	Wednesday
Breakfast: **Snack-1:** **Lunch:** **Snack-2:** **Dinner:** **Snack-3:** **Drinks:**	**Breakfast:** **Snack-1:** **Lunch:** **Snack-2:** **Dinner:** **Snack-3:** **Drinks:**
Thursday	Thursday
Breakfast: **Snack-1:** **Lunch:** **Snack-2:** **Dinner:** **Snack-3:** **Drinks:**	**Breakfast:** **Snack-1:** **Lunch:** **Snack-2:** **Dinner:** **Snack-3:** **Drinks:**
Friday	Friday
Breakfast: **Snack-1:** **Lunch:** **Snack-2:** **Dinner:** **Snack-3:** **Drinks:**	**Breakfast:** **Snack-1:** **Lunch:** **Snack-2:** **Dinner:** **Snack-3:** **Drinks:**
Saturday	Saturday
Breakfast: **Snack-1:** **Lunch:** **Snack-2:** **Dinner:** **Snack-3:** **Drinks:**	**Breakfast:** **Snack-1:** **Lunch:** **Snack-2:** **Dinner:** **Snack-3:** **Drinks:**
Sunday	Sunday
Breakfast: **Snack-1:** **Lunch:** **Snack-2:** **Dinner:** **Snack-3:** **Drinks:**	**Breakfast:** **Snack-1:** **Lunch:** **Snack-2:** **Dinner:** **Snack-3:** **Drinks:**

This book aimed to provide you with useful information about low fructose healthy nutritional choices, food preparation, how to cook for fructose intolerant people and essential dietary tips you need to follow to effectively manage the fructose intolerance. It also guided you through meal planning and how to create biweekly cooking plans.

Comprehensive lists of foods to avoid and foods to each for people with fructose intolerance presented in Chapter 1, and Chapter 2 suggested essential tips for food preparation and meal planning. You learned more than 120 different cooking recipes presented in Chapter 3 of this book, including cooking tips and fructose intolerance-related tips.

Chapter 4 presented biweekly cooking plan samples. The blanked biweekly cooking plan tables in this chapter can be used by you to write your own cooking plans. Remember that it is always essential to talk to your doctor about suggested foods or any recommended diets you would like to follow.

Now, you have learned the basics of the fructose free diet, food preparation, and meal plans by reading this book. If you found out that you would like to have a comprehensive journal or diary that has been designed explicitly for IBS patients to record all your Fructose Intolerance-related history, you may want to take a look at the following book in the amazon store prepared by the same author of this book:

Low FODMAP Journal, Specifically Designed for Irritable Bowel Syndrome (IBS) Patients, by Monet Manbacci, P.h.D., Available in Amazon Paperback Format, Jan. 2020.

About The Author

Monet Manbacci, Ph.D., is the author of *"Low FODMAP Comprehensive Diet Guide and Cookbook"*, *"Crohn's Disease Comprehensive diet guide and cookbook"*, *"The Comprehensive Guide to Crohn's Disease"*, *"Ulcerative Colitis Comprehensive Diet Guide and Cookbook"*, and *"Low Fodmap Journal: Specifically Designed for Irritable Bowel Syndrome (IBS) Patients"* Books. He is an IBD patient initially diagnosed with IBS, who has a Doctor of Philosophy (Ph.D.) degree in Applied Sciences and has been involved in academic and scientific research for more than 14 years.

OTHER BOOKS BY HEALTHVIEW PUBLISHERS:

Low FODMAP Journal, Specifically Designed for Irritable Bowel Syndrome (IBS) Patients, by Monet Manbacci, P.h.D., Available in Amazon Paperback Format, Jan. 2020.

Crohn's Disease Comprehensive Diet Guide and Cookbook, by Monet Manbacci, P.h.D., Available in Amazon Kindle & Paperback Formats, 2019.

Ulcerative Colitis Comprehensive Diet Guide and Cookbook, by Monet Manbacci, P.h.D., Available in Amazon Kindle & Paperback Formats, 2020.

The Comprehensive Guide to Crohn's Disease, All You Need to Know About Crohn's Disease, from Diagnosis to Management & Treatment, by Monet Manbacci, P.h.D., Available in Amazon Kindle & Paperback Formats, 2019.

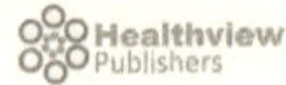